Infla-Menses:
The Connection Between Inflammation
and Menstrual Problems

Infla-Menses:
The Connection Between Inflammation and Menstrual Problems

Alexandra Preston

Alexandra Preston
2019

First Printing: 2019

ISBN 978-0-646-81139-0

www.alexandra-springnaturalhealth.com

Ordering Information:
Special discounts are available on quantity purchases by corporations, associations, educators, and others. For details, contact the publisher at the above listed address.

U.S. trade bookstores and wholesalers: Please contact Alexandra Preston through her website, or by email at alexandra.p.naturopath@protonmail.com.

Dedication

To all of my friends and family who have supported me;
to Ruth Elisabeth, for helping me find my voice; to Ira
Pastor, who helped me name this book; and to Dr Ursula
Jacob, for the publication that first inspired me.

Contents

Starter Recipes for an Anti-Inflammatory Diet ... 184

Appendix: Diet Diary and Cycle Chart ... 212

References ... 219

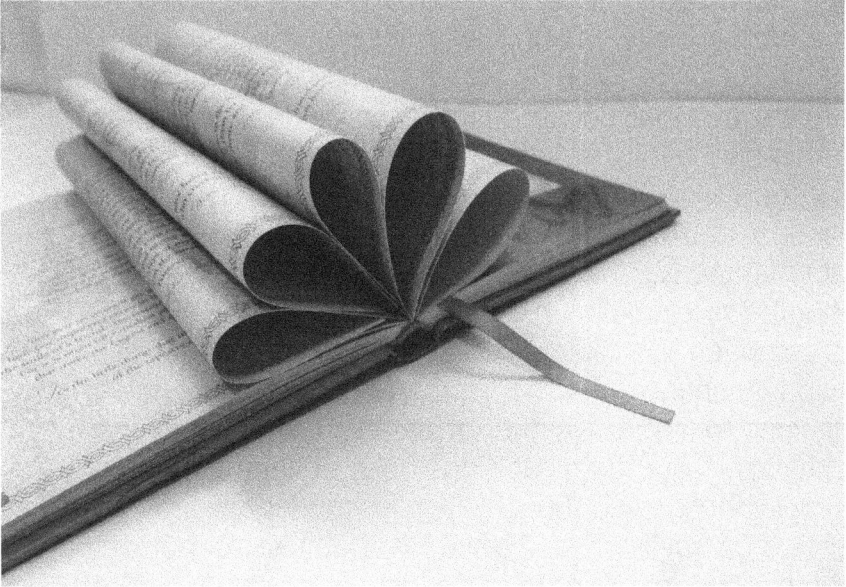

My Experience

This book is for women who, as I once did, wonder what they're missing when it comes to achieving optimal health and a menstrual cycle that won't hold them back. It's also for women who know that they deserve better than to "put up with it" every month, whether it be as patient or carer. You may be reading it for yourself, a loved one, because you want to pursue a career in holistic health, or all of the above. So why did I decide to break free from the long-suffering-woman mould, heal myself and eventually write this book?

For seven years, from when I was 13 until I was 20, I struggled almost every month with often debilitating period pain that stopped me from going to school or work for at least part of the day. Why seven years – including for half of my naturopathy degree? The emphasis on hormonal health meant that I couldn't find the right treatment. Herbal remedies focusing on hormone balance only had minimal effects, and PMS-focused information didn't apply to me (when you get no emotional symptoms, but everything insists you do, you end up resenting your cycle even more!). Analgesics like cramp bark didn't work either, and the effects of pharmaceutical pain relief stopped quickly – it never took long for me to build up a tolerance to them. I never tried prescription painkillers because I value and need a clear mind. Acupuncture had a temporary effect, and it never seemed to matter whether or not I ate soy. I would be exhausted, but red meat didn't help; neither did iron supplements, even though I always tended towards a heavy flow. I had belly danced since I was almost 14, but despite the positive results others got, that didn't seem to relieve anything either, unless it prevented things from getting worse.

Sometimes, even teachers said that I'd have to "put up with it" or have a baby! Grr! If anyone pressures you to have a baby, or insists that it is the only way to solve a problem, run! Motherhood should always be a free choice – not a forced choice, not an obligation. Coming into womanhood is an open-ended story; it's not about enduring things you don't want such as health complaints. Realising this, in fact, helped a little with preventing cramps; my first advice to you is to reject the idea that being a woman means restrictions, being pushed into certain roles and suffering. Just as you have a right to education, to provide for yourself and to make your own decisions, you have the right to optimal health.

It was by chance that I read an article by Dr Ursula Jacob from Germany, on fermented soy for autoimmune disease. Because of this, combined with our college teachers' urging that we eat fermented foods every day, I decided to start eating miso paste as a broth on a daily basis. To my surprise, I had little to no cramping on my next period! I also quit gluten, which helped to balance my immune system and relieve other inflammatory issues. As miso is very salty and I was about to travel to Europe for a month, I eventually switched to a turmeric supplement for convenience, with even better results. Over time, I started to get lighter periods and the fatigue that once felt crushing started to lift, especially when I would take B vitamins. My problem was inflammation, as it had been since I was a young child when I had asthma and allergies. Now, I know that I can only keep my own menstrual difficulties away (or at least mostly out of my hair) by ensuring that my levels of inflammation are low enough.

The Menstrual Cycle and Inflammation

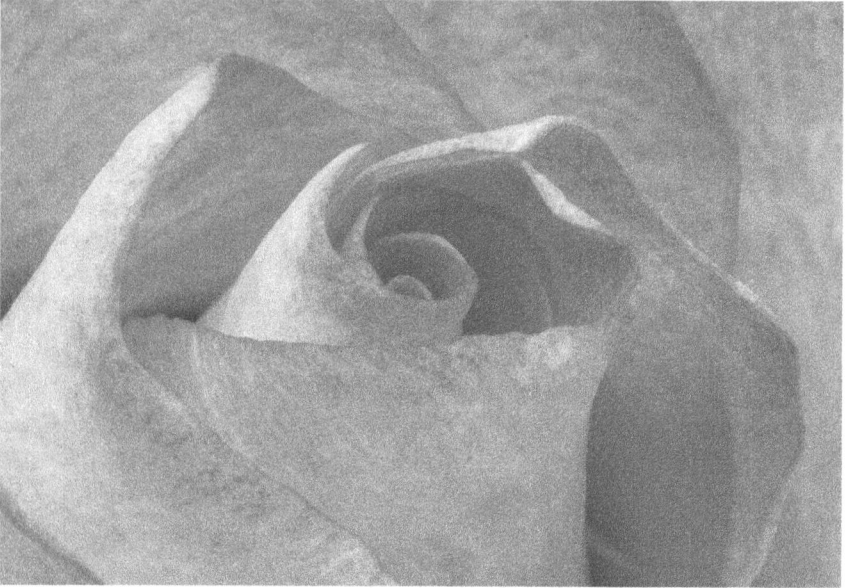

Menstruation depends on a functioning hormonal feedback system, along with a sufficient number of eggs in the ovaries. The menstrual cycle turns on when the hypothalamus secretes a hormone called gonadotrophin-releasing hormone (GnRH), which instructs the pituitary gland to produce follicular stimulating hormone (FSH). FSH stimulates growth of around 20-30 eggs per cycle; these produce oestrogen and trigger a surge of luteinising hormone (LH). This surge in turn causes ovulation, where the dominant egg is released. The oestrogen meanwhile stimulates growth of the uterine lining, and progesterone (plus more oestrogen) is produced by the egg's follicle once it leaves for the Fallopian tubes. If there is no pregnancy, the follicle stops producing progesterone and oestrogen, causing the breakdown of the lining and therefore menstruation. It's a cycle of coming and passing, much like that of flowers. A normal menstrual cycle ranges from 21-35 days in length, with 4-7 days of bleeding time. Two, or even up to nine, days can be normal and healthy for you too, where 30-40mL or even up to 80mL of "blood" is lost. Calling menstrual flow "blood" is common and easier to say (and read!), but not entirely accurate; most of the flow is broken down uterine lining, with only one third of it being actual blood. Ovulation typically happens around mid-cycle at day 14, but the normal range is from day 10 to 16.

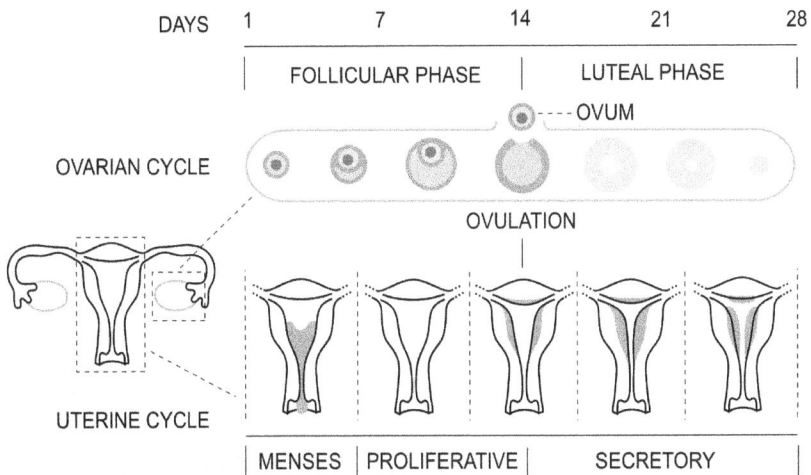

Figure 1: The phases of the menstrual cycle. Source: Isometrik and Kaldari (CC by S.A.: 3.0)

Period Pain

Period pain is sadly common among girls and younger women. Simply put, it is caused by the normal contractions of the uterus, which are necessary to expel the old lining, coming on too strong. We don't notice mild contractions, but overstimulated uterine muscle, heavy flow or clotting can make them stronger.

Between 50% and 80% of women with a menstrual cycle are estimated to suffer from primary dysmenorrhoea, and in teenage girls this ranges from 20-90% depending on the population surveyed. Primary dysmenorrhoea is the medical term for period pain that isn't caused by a disease like endometriosis or fibroids. It is called secondary dysmenorrhoea if it came from one or more of these diseases. The risk of "primary" period pain rises until the age of 20, and it appears during the first six months to two years after the menstrual cycle starts.

It is no secret that inflammation is a key contributor, and often driver, of period pain and other menstrual problems. The major inflammatory chemicals produced by the body in cases of period pain are products of what are known as the cyclo-oxygenase (COX) and lipoxygenase (LOX) pathways, the "children" of an inflammatory fatty acid known as arachidonic acid. Prostaglandins and thromboxanes belong to COX; the HETEs and leukotrienes belong to LOX. Women with period pain are more likely to have these inflammatory chemicals in their menstrual blood at higher levels than women who are pain-free, but 12-HETE is the most strongly associated. You can remember it by thinking of "HETE" as

6

"heat", because inflammation often features a heat sensation.

The most widely known inflammatory cause of period pain is an imbalance of the prostaglandins, thanks to the ubiquitous evening primrose oil supplements (more on that later). Some increase inflammation, while others resolve it. The two main prostaglandins involved in period pain are abbreviated as PGF2 and PGE2, which are produced from arachidonic acid. They cause the contractions in the uterus in order to help break down and remove the old lining. To make matters worse, at high enough levels they increase muscle contractions in the stomach, meaning that nausea and vomiting can accompany period pain.

Treatments aimed at relieving inflammation work by reducing or re-balancing chemicals such as the prostaglandins; we need some of all of these so our immune cells can communicate with the rest of the body and each other. Still keeping up? I'm explaining these technical terms now, because the different remedies for period pain, heavy flow and PMS have their own sets of pathways that they work on, so you will be seeing these names later. You may also be reading this because you want to enter a career in the health industry, or because you are a carer or patient advocate for someone seeking true healing and recovery from an illness or injury. In any case, understanding the science is important, and yes, I do explain the physiology behind the treatments I recommend during consultations.

Premenstrual Syndrome (PMS)

PMS is also a very common complaint, with 85% of women reporting one or more symptoms. Sadly, 7% experience symptoms so debilitating that their daily activities are limited. There are around 150 possible symptoms of PMS, so every woman who gets it is different. Common psychological problems include anxiety, anger, irritability and poor concentration; physical issues can include fatigue, headaches, carbohydrate cravings, breast tenderness and water retention. For many years, PMS has often gone unrecognised by healthcare professionals, because its symptoms, signs and treatment are so different for every patient. There are, however, several common symptom clusters:

PMS Type	Common Symptom Clusters
PMS-A (Anxiety)	Anxiety, crying, emotionality, mood swings, nervousness, paranoia, tension
PMS-C (Cravings)	Cravings, especially for sugar or chocolate; fatigue; headaches; hypoglycaemia; increased appetite
PMS-D (Depression)	Depression, confusion, insomnia, poor memory, withdrawal. Seek immediate help if you feel at risk.
PMS-H (Hydration/Headache)	Fluid retention, bloating, sore breasts, weight gain
PMS-P (Pain)	Pain in the abdomen, back or joints, headache

Inflammation is also linked to PMS. In a study of almost three thousand women from 2015, researchers compared levels of an inflammatory marker known as high-sensitivity C-reactive protein (hs-CRP) to the presence of PMS symptoms. This is a common marker to measure, as it's readily accessible by blood test and rises and falls rapidly in response to inflammation. The others I mentioned earlier aren't so often tested. Greater hs-CRP levels were associated with around a 27% higher risk of mood symptoms or breast pain, and a 40% higher risk of abdominal cramps, back pain, cravings, weight gain and bloating. Obesity and smoking were also linked to a greater risk of PMS symptoms, as they cause inflammation. This study involved women aged 42-52 of diverse ethnic backgrounds; others showing weaker associations typically had younger, white women.

A smaller but comprehensive study on 277 young women focused on measuring a wide range of the immune-signalling interleukins, and compared them to 26 physical and mental symptoms of PMS. These included cramps, cravings, anxiety, irritability, bloating, constipation, acne and headaches. They were asked to indicate if they had experienced each symptom for most months of the year, for at least several days before their periods began, and to rate each from 1 (no symptom) to 4 (severe). Other questions were how much their symptoms affected their daily lives in areas such as work or personal relationships. Around 22% of the women had very little to no PMS symptoms, and were used as a control group for comparison. The only significant difference between the women with PMS and the control group was that their smoking rates were much higher: 32.4% of them had ever smoked, compared to 9% of those who didn't have

Infla-Menses

PMS. Several interleukins were much higher in women with PMS; sometimes even more than double that of the control group. Interestingly, the most commonly studied inflammatory markers (CRP, TNF-a, IL-1b and IL-6) were not really linked to PMS. Some other studies this book references did find associations, but everyone is different in terms of how and why inflammation causes health problems. The interleukins that *were* related, however, haven't been so extensively researched for their effects on women's health issues or mental health.

Perhaps the most well-known (or most infamous) symptom of PMS is mood dysregulation, which can affect our relationships, careers and overall quality of life. A study on female soccer players found that those with PMS had higher levels of depression if their levels of IL-10, an anti-inflammatory interleukin, were lower. Pre-game, they reported greater tension in the follicular phase and more depression in the luteal phase than women without PMS. After the game, their levels of IL-6, which is pro-inflammatory, fell regardless of what menstrual cycle phase they were in.

Premenstrual Dysphoric Disorder (PMDD)

If mood dysregulation is severe, you may have PMDD. Depression, a prominent feature of PMDD, is linked to a dysregulated immune system and inflammation. We think of it as a chemical imbalance originating in the brain, but its true cause is often inflammation which disrupts neurotransmitter production. Neurotransmitters are chemicals produced by the brain to aid communication.

Some regulate mood, some stimulate certain functions, and others still provide a calming effect to prevent overexcitement.

Both PMDD and major depressive disorder (MDD) have inflammation as an underlying cause. Inflammation even raises your risk of developing depression in the future, so you're better off knocking it on the head *now* than later. Production of some inflammatory markers is higher in the luteal phase, with levels of these markers related to the severity of pre-menstrual symptom scores in women with no chronic illnesses. The treatments discussed in the review that this paragraph references mostly consist of antidepressants, hormone therapies and psychotherapies. If the root cause of your issues is inflammation, these will only address the symptoms, at best.

Inflammation leads to another mechanism behind depression: an impairment of the ability to produce new neurons, something once thought to be impossible. In MDD, which can be tied to severe PMS, stem cells in the brain do not divide as much before starting to become neurons, and their survival rates are lower. We see this in the reduced volume of the hippocampus, the main memory centre of the brain, and the impaired memory and learning that people with depression know far too well. A friend I was once close with sadly dropped out of our naturopathy degree largely because of this, and her illness damaged our relationship. Treatments that have an antidepressant effect by affecting the levels of neurotransmitters can, fortunately, raise the rate of brain regeneration back to normal levels. If we couldn't produce new neurons, learning and memory would be (at the very least) difficult, and dementias would strike earlier and more often. In fact, Dr Dale Bredesen writes in *The End of Alzheimer's* that many cases of the disease feature inflammation as one of the root causes, which partly acts by impairing these normal regeneration processes.

Fatigue

Fatigue, a common occurrence during menstruation, is also at least partly tied to inflammation. In fact, research has reported that 85% of women who suffer from dysmenorrhoea have fatigue too. Most acute and chronic inflammatory diseases feature the symptom, which will not improve with rest. The level of inflammatory markers in the blood is often related to the severity of fatigue, while resolving it improves energy. These markers disrupt the production and function of certain hormones that play important roles in energy metabolism. Additionally, iron levels are depleted in cases of chronic inflammation, causing anaemia. Many women will tell you to just stop and rest during your period, but isn't it better to relieve fatigue at its cause? Resting all day for a few days is not always an option, such as if it's a hectic time at work, exam week, or you're on holiday.

Menorrhagia

Menorrhagia, the medical term for a heavy flow, is defined as over 80mL of menstrual fluid being passed per month. It can be part of another condition such as endometriosis or fibroids. However, you may still have trouble with above-average flow that doesn't meet these criteria and is not a symptom of disease such as endometriosis. Menorrhagia is caused by both hormonal imbalances and inflammation, in particular through the prostaglandin pathways. Sometimes, vitamin K deficiency is behind it, as well as clotting disorders (get tested if you have severe, unresponsive menorrhagia).

Heavy bleeding can also cause clots, as the normal anti-clotting factors in the uterus cannot always keep up. A heavy flow involves the process of new blood vessel growth occurring to excess. We need it for normal tissue regeneration and maintenance, but too much means more uterine lining will be built up. It is controlled by both growth factors – a type of "signal" that tells our cells what to do – and inflammation. When I began to control my own inflammation, my periods became lighter. Sadly, surveys have shown that the majority of women with menorrhagia believe they just have to live with it.

Menstrual Migraine

A menstrual migraine is a migraine that occurs either during menstruation, or within three days before it begins. Over half of women who suffer from migraines report an association with menstruation. Population studies show that women are at their highest risk of attack during or just before their periods, and are at their lowest risk around ovulation. Conventional treatment is often the same as that for general migraines, but sometimes it involves hormonal interventions to smooth out the peaks and dips in sex hormones that naturally occur across our cycles.

Migraine attacks are also linked to inflammation and related issues, in at least some cases. Chronic pain disorders, including migraine, may be linked with changes to the blood-brain barrier (BBB). Inflammatory pain changes structures of transporter proteins in the barrier, and activates cells that are kind of like security guards for the brain. Peripheral inflammation also increases the level of zonulin – that protein affected by gluten in the intestines which allows it to cause leaky gut – and reduces occludin, which keeps the BBB closed to many unfriendly substances.

Additionally, a type of protein known as matrix metalloprotease has been found in higher levels among women with migraines. These are meant to aid tissue rebuilding after acute injury, but in chronic illness they cause trouble by letting inflammatory responses in and allowing inappropriate cellular migration. During a migraine attack, research points to a sort of "breakdown" or permeability increase in the BBB. Barrier breakdown may even result in lasting "pain behaviour" – let's break the cycle ASAP!

Endometriosis

Endometriosis, where the uterine lining grows in other areas of the body, causes extreme examples of period pain, heavy bleeding and PMS. It is a common cause of secondary dysmenorrhoea, as it affects 6-10% of younger (reproductive age) women. Because most women (76-90%) do have uterine lining cells present outside the uterus, the theory of retrograde menstruation – where it flows backwards – is incomplete without looking at its link with inflammation and disruption of the immune system. Women with this condition are more likely to also have other inflammatory diseases, such as rheumatoid arthritis, thyroid disorders, lupus, or multiple sclerosis, than women who don't have it.

Endometriosis is best treated with an integrative approach, and many natural interventions do overlap with those for primary pain, PMS and milder cases of menorrhagia.

Endometriosis is most likely a combination of hormonal imbalances and inflammation interacting with each other. Expression of oestrogen receptors on the macrophages, a type of immune cell, is linked to the amount of inflammatory substances they produce. An increase in oestrogen levels also raises COX-2 expression. Additionally, a stress hormone known as corticotrophin-releasing hormone (CRH) has been shown to worsen the peritoneal inflammation seen in endometriosis (this means in the abdominal cavity, but outside the organs).

The theory of retrograde menstruation is quite old – one of the first works discussing it was published in 1927! More recently, high-tech methods of analysis have found that inflammation likely contributes to endometriosis. Inflammatory mediators such as TNF-a, IL-6 and IL-1b are shown to have activity in endometriosis, and inflammation is known to impair blood vessel function in the disease. Biopsies have also shown that some types of immune cells are more reactive, particularly in stage III and IV endometriosis; stage IV is the most severe form. However, the T-suppressor cells, which dampen down the immune response, are shown to be decreased, while the types of T cells involved in promoting this inflammatory immune response are present in higher numbers and are more active.

What's more, women with endometriosis are documented to have higher levels of lipopolysaccharides (LPS) in menstrual and peritoneal fluid than healthy women.

Infla-Menses

These are toxins produced by bacteria; if they get into the bloodstream, they increase inflammation and endometrial tissue overgrowth. They make their way into the bloodstream through dysbiosis and leaky gut. This finding helps to explain the high prevalence of Irritable Bowel Syndrome (IBS) in women with endometriosis – up to 80% of sufferers also have the syndrome. To be specific, researchers found a considerable presence of *E. coli*, which may be caused by both leaky gut and poor hygiene.

Polycystic Ovarian Syndrome (PCOS)

Polycystic Ovarian Syndrome (PCOS) is a tangled mess of hormone imbalances which leads to menstrual problems, ovarian cysts and often infertility. Abnormal GnRH secretion causes high luteinising hormone, which stimulates the ovaries and their production of sex hormones, while insulin resistance produces even more oestrogen, testosterone and growth factors. High DHEAS from the adrenal glands and aromatase, an enzyme that produces oestrogen from testosterone, don't help either.

PCOS is linked to metabolic syndrome, which now affects one in four adults and one in ten teenagers! This is a cluster of obesity, especially abdominal fat; high blood sugar, 5.6mmol/L or over; high blood pressure and dysregulated blood lipids, usually low HDL and high triglycerides. With inflammatory immune chemicals being produced at a higher level with excess body fat, inflammation plays a key role in metabolic syndrome and related issues like PCOS. Those produced by fat are known as adipokines. Consequences of inflammation, such as damage to the small blood vessels, may contribute to insulin resistance too.

Research specifically on PCOS has found that it is associated with multiple markers of inflammation, along with damage to the blood vessels and oxidative stress. A diet high in sugar and unhealthy fats was shown to cause leaky gut in women with PCOS, which allows inflammatory chemicals made by bacteria into the bloodstream. This can overstimulate the immune system so it overreacts and starts to work against insulin receptors.

Uterine Fibroids

Uterine fibroids are a common occurrence, with up to half of all women developing them at some point in their lives. Most do not cause symptoms, and they often shrink during menopause when oestrogen levels fall. When they do cause symptoms, these include a general feeling of heaviness, abdominal enlargement, backache, infertility, miscarriage, painful urination, menorrhagia and dysmenorrhoea. Some women can suffer from a torrential flow, and are so worried about flooding that they stay home on their heaviest days. Fibroids can become so detrimental to our health and quality of life that they are actually the leading indication for hysterectomy, costing $6 billion per year in the United States alone. It is far better to address them in their earlier stages as they are difficult to shrink.

Fibroids themselves are not hormonally active, but are hyper-responsive to oestrogen. The connection between oestrogen and inflammation is the enzyme aromatase, which

Infla-Menses

is increased by the inflammatory PGE2 and converts testosterone (yes, women need a small amount of this!) to oestrogen. Obesity is another major contributor to fibroids, with women weighing over 70kg having triple the risk compared to women who weigh under 50kg. This is far below the ideal weight for many women, however; look at body composition and BMI instead of just a number. High body fat not only increases the level of aromatase, but also lowers sex hormone-binding globulin (SHBG), which raises the level of active oestrogen.

Besides aromatase and the E2 prostaglandins, there are other inflammatory factors behind fibroids. Inflammation contributes to their cell proliferation and formation of new blood vessels, which is necessary for their continued growth. This may be triggered by an altered response to harmful stimuli, such as impaired oxygen flow, tissue injury or toxin exposure. The cyclo-oxygenase-2 (COX-2) pathway has been found to influence fibroid development, and so has the NF-kB pathway.

Fibrosis, a feature of many inflammatory diseases, is also present in fibroids, hence their name. The fibrotic tissue may in turn contribute to the continuation of inflammation, by serving as a storage space for inflammatory mediators, growth factors and mediators involved in blood vessel growth, creating a nasty cycle. One non-sex hormone growth factor linked with fibroids is IGF-1, which is raised by many inflammatory foods. Oxidative stress contributes to their growth too, with the cells in fibroids containing lower levels of antioxidant enzymes compared to normal uterine cells. Fat cells play their role by producing TNF-a, an inflammatory mediator that boosts fibroid development.

Alexandra Preston

Adjunctive Treatment for Pelvic Inflammatory Disease

Pelvic Inflammatory Disease (PID) is a serious, acute condition triggered by infection. In every case, you would need antimicrobial treatment to kill off the bacteria, but anti-inflammatories can speed healing and reduce the risk of long-term effects. Here, pain is constant, on both sides, and worsened by exercise. It must be examined to rule out other conditions such as appendicitis or ectopic pregnancy, and will stand out from usual symptoms. If this sounds like you, see a doctor as soon as possible for a correct diagnosis.

Two examples of anti-inflammatory adjunctive treatments are bromelain and vitamin C, which can help to prevent scarring, but the best prevention is hygiene. Loss of the cervical plug during menstruation increases the risk of STDs leading to PID; this is probably how the cultural taboo against period sex originated. Barrier methods of contraception are essential, preferably condoms and especially if you aren't in a long-term, monogamous relationship.

Other Inflammatory Conditions

Unlike many others on women's health, this book comes from an antiaging, or longevity-promoting, angle instead of fertility. We all have a life, a body, and know people who are just irreplaceable in our lives, but not everyone wants a baby. Some do not want children yet, while other women are childfree for life. The other reason why I am focusing on inflammation is that while acute inflammation is necessary to fight infection and stimulate healing, chronic inflammation

Infla-Menses

causes tissue damage and disrupts immunity. It's a main driver of the aging process, and many chronic illnesses such as cardiovascular disease, neurological disorders (e.g. dementia), diabetes and arthritis. You may be only 18 years old, for example, but it's better to start preventing illnesses and putting everything in place to live as long and healthy as you can now rather than later.

Many chronic health problems also worsen at certain times of the menstrual cycle, and if you're trying to heal from them or stay in remission, this could be a significant setback. These include acne, IBS, rheumatoid arthritis, diabetes, asthma, multiple sclerosis, bipolar disorder and even epilepsy, which can all worsen at certain times. For example, up to 40% of asthmatic women get worse before their periods start. Many women who have conditions such as inflammatory bowel disease (IBD) or gingivitis suffer from a worsening of symptoms in the premenstrual or menstrual stage of their cycles. Part of this is because hormonal fluctuations also affect immune and neuroendocrine balance. Even if you do have a confirmed hormone imbalance, it is important to address the problem from both ends by healing hormonal issues and inflammation.

Why does this happen? Oestrogen affects the development and behaviour of immune cells, but precisely how depends on the individual. How you detoxify old oestrogen; whether your immune system is reacting to your own tissues or an external source, such as a food intolerance or chronic infection; what organs or tissues are affected; and differences in oestrogen receptors and immune function determine whether oestrogen is pro- or anti-inflammatory for you.

Many immune responses can be divided into two categories depending on what type of T-helper cell is predominately involved: Th-1 or Th-2. The T-helper cells play an essential role in fighting off invaders, and also sadly things they have been led to think are a problem, such as foods, fur or even ourselves! The luteal phase (after ovulation) is associated with a shift to Th-2 dominant immune responses, for example. This can help to relieve symptoms of problems linked to Th-1 dominance, but worsen illnesses tied to Th-2 dominance. Again, balance is the key.

Central hypersensitivity is a particularly nasty way that inflammation can affect the menstrual cycle and our overall health. This is when inflammation and/or direct damage to the nervous system lowers our pain threshold, which can lead to chronic pain conditions if not reversed. The COX-2 pathway, also involved in dysmenorrhoea, is triggered in a certain type of neuron, leading to PGE2 production. PGE2 then increases the pain response and prevents the normal inhibitory response that would otherwise stop the nervous system from overreacting. When this mechanism was removed from neurons in lab experiments, the hypersensitive reaction was no more, even though the overall inflammatory response in other areas of the body continued. To make things worse, chronic inflammation can "teach" the microglia – a type of neuron that acts as the brain and spinal cord's immune system – to continue the response.

The "classic" central hypersensitivity disorder is fibromyalgia, but it also includes dysmenorrhoea, IBS, migraine, chronic fatigue syndrome, restless legs syndrome and rheumatoid arthritis. In some cases where your symptoms worsen at certain times but are present all month long, the residual problems may be from central hypersensitivity. You need to relieve the inflammatory response in order to help re-train the nervous system to behave normally. Inflammation and psychosocial causes such as trauma, abuse and how you learnt to deal with stress are commonly seen together in these disorders. One of my own clients with IBS not only had to heal their gut, but also from their history of abuse.

If you have a chronic illness, such as IBS, IBD, fibromyalgia, arthritis or anything else, track everything for at least one cycle either before you get started on healing or when you've just begun, in order to understand where the problem is coming from. There are plenty of menstrual cycle tracking apps out there, or you can write everything in a diary if you (like me) prefer something physical and more free-form. I also have a cycle chart in the Appendix for you to photocopy and fill out.

It isn't just about clinically diagnosable diseases, either. Stopping chronic inflammation in its tracks helps to promote overall health and wellbeing wherever you are on your cycle, before any disease process may manifest. Researchers have even found that reducing chronic inflammation helps our stem cells to survive and aid healing, through ways such as directly turning into specific cell types. Yes, it's not mad science, the stem cell therapies you may hear about being trialled are just amplifying a natural process! Even during everyday wear and tear, such as when you're playing sport or working out, your stem cells are busy repairing microscopic damage.

Alexandra Preston

The advantage of having a menstrual cycle is that it acts as a monthly(ish) report card for your internal health. A month is enough time for the effects of your diet, lifestyle and supplements, if any, to build up, but not so long that it takes seemingly forever to be rewarded for healthier habits. Finally, don't worry that living longer means spending more years in poor health! All truly life-extending interventions, including quitting smoking and moderate exercise, work by fighting aging and preventing illness. On the other hand, a drop in life expectancy is a sign of degeneration on some level – quality and quantity are truly inseparable in this case.

What Causes Inflammation?

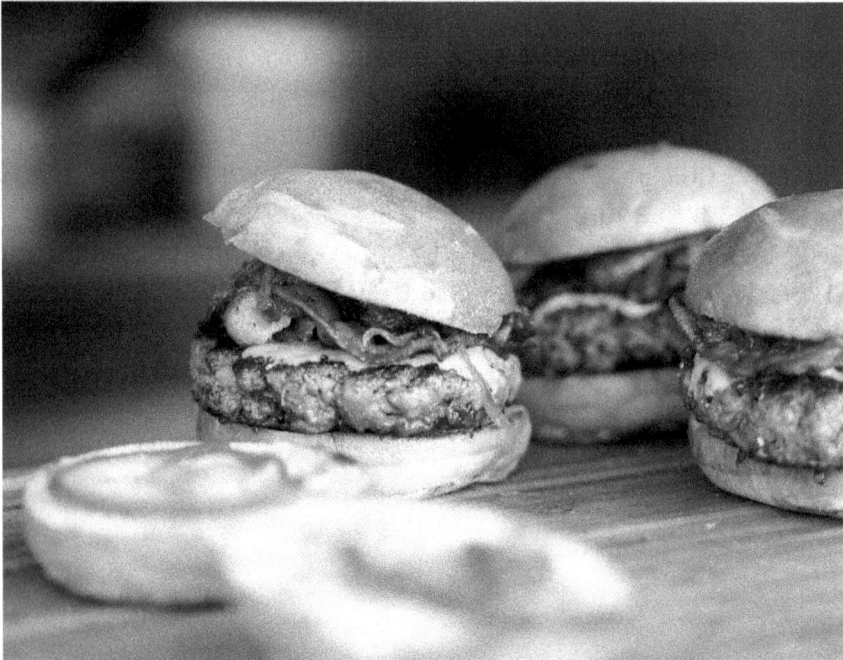

For a healthy, trouble-free menstrual cycle, it's important to reduce or eliminate our exposure to triggers of inflammation. Your tolerance to any of these depends on individual factors; it's the same for your ideal weight and ability to tolerate toxins. You may be able to tolerate some of these as part of your regular diet, or there may be some you must strictly avoid. Everyone is different. Let's start with what is fast becoming an infamous dietary pattern.

Dietary Factors

The Modern Western Diet

While European cultures are all considered part of the West, it is important to differentiate between healthy traditional Western cuisines and the unhealthy pattern that emerged from some regions. What we define as the modern Western diet is high in red and processed meat, sugary foods, refined grains, dairy, white potatoes, trans fats and processed foods.

In *The End of Alzheimer's*, Dr Bredesen likes to call an especially dangerous trio of foods the "Berfooda Triangle", all too common in the modern Western diet. This is a combination of simple carbs, lack of fibre and saturated fat – a cheeseburger, chips (fries) and a soft drink or milkshake. Saturated fats aren't bad alone and in moderation, but are inflammatory with sugar and no fibre. A lack of fibre also speeds carbohydrate absorption, which increases inflammation through advanced glycation end-products (AGES) and a rapid spike in insulin.

Women in the Nurses' Health Study following this pattern had higher levels of inflammatory markers, such as CRP and IL-6, compared to those eating more fruits, vegetables, legumes, wholegrains, fish and poultry. Fruit and vegetables reduce inflammation by their antioxidant effects, as oxidative stress turns on the NF-kB pathway. Wholegrains beat refined grains because they have more fibre, vitamins, minerals and phytochemicals. Refined grains also make blood sugar and insulin rise too rapidly after eating them.

Infla-Menses

If you are reading because you or someone you love has PCOS, the modern Western diet has more harmful effects. The liver deals with four things that aren't insulin regulated and don't have an appropriate "off switch" for excessive amounts, which leads to an increase in body fat. These are trans fats, alcohol, fructose and the branch-chained amino acids (BCAAs). The BCAAs are necessary for muscle growth and are highest in meat, but don't eat too much! If you do eat meat, keep it anywhere from once a day to once a week. All of these four food components are featured too prominently in the modern Western diet, in meat; alcoholic drinks; margarine and other processed foods; and soft drinks as high-fructose corn syrup (HCFS).

Do you have depression, or care about someone who does? A large review totalling 101,950 participants set out to determine if such an inflammatory diet increases the risk of this disease. What were the results? Across a wide range of ages and countries, it was associated with a 40% higher rate of depression. Features of an inflammatory diet that the researchers highlighted include lower consumption of wholegrains, flavonoids and choline-containing foods. These include cauliflower, broccoli and eggs. The link between inflammatory foods and depression goes both ways, as mental or emotional pain often leads people to consume unhealthy foods.

It isn't about the unhealthy lifestyle choices that often accompany this eating pattern, either. In a laboratory study, the mouse equivalent of the Western diet was shown to disrupt immune function. The diet caused systemic inflammation that resolved once they were given their usual diet, but their immune cells were still over-responsive once provoked. Even after four weeks of the healthier diet, they stayed hyperactive. If your level of inflammation is more severe, such as if you have been diagnosed with an autoimmune disease, this unfortunately means that an occasional forbidden treat must stay exactly that – forbidden. In less serious cases, you may be able to get away with that meat pie or hot dog if you get right back into an anti-inflammatory eating pattern (go to the Golden Milk recipe for a DIY supplement if you need an extra helping hand). The Western diet was found to cause inflammation by changing the expression of genes in a way that hyped up the immune response. The immune system kept this expression pattern in a similar way to how it remembers when you've been exposed to a virus or bacteria before; its intent is to protect you from the "infection", even if it's just the wrong foods.

Why do so many people in the nutrition world criticise the Western diet, and why does my recipe list at the end of this book contain so many non-Western foods? It is scientifically proven that Western food, especially Anglo-Western food, is bland. A study in *Nature* showed a higher rate of shared flavour compounds in North American cuisine and a greater reliance on wheat, dairy and eggs, compared to the diverse, more plant-based Asian cuisines. While some traditional Western diets are just plain boring, like the boil-everything-and-what-are-spices old English cuisine, the modern Western diet is even worse for your health. Apparently the solution to a lack of colour and flavour was simply to increase the amount of meat, refined grains, sugar, dairy and artificial food ingredients. European cuisines from the Mediterranean, however, have more colour and flavour to them, and a greater proportion of proteins and fats coming from anti-inflammatory sources.

Red Meat

Red meat has received increased attention for its environmental impact in recent years, particularly in the case of beef, which uses up to 168 times more land than plant foods and over 20 times that of other terrestrial animal products. However, red meat can cause menstrual difficulties in many women too. It contains high levels of arachidonic acid, the precursor to inflammatory prostaglandins, and may be linked to endometriosis because of this.

A 22-year-long study of almost 82,000 women found that those who ate two or more servings of red meat every day(!) had a 56% higher risk of the disease, compared to women only eating it once per week or less. This link was stronger for non-processed meat and for women who were not infertile. Processed meats, i.e. sausages and other things we joke about not being all meat, were only associated with a 20% increased risk. Poultry (chicken, turkey etc.), fish, shellfish, and eggs were not linked with the development of endometriosis. However, poultry, pork and eggs do contain considerable amounts of arachidonic acid, so don't eat them to excess. As eggs are very nutrient-dense, I would not recommend avoiding them unless you really want to be vegan and have done your research.

Whether or not it is processed, red meat is linked to a higher endometriosis risk. Replacing it with fish, eggs or shellfish is related to a lower chance of developing it, but eating more poultry may put you at a greater risk of endometriosis too (though not as much as red meat).This is partly due to the inflammatory fats, as a diet high in these can also contribute to endometriosis even if there is no weight gain, insulin resistance or ovarian dysfunction. But doesn't red meat also cause endometriosis by raising oestrogen? Actually, blood levels of oestradiol are similar in women with and without the disease, but it may still be a contributing factor to problems in endometrial and endometriotic tissue.

Other research has shown a link between meat intake and primary dysmenorrhoea. Although numbers of vegetarian women were too small to reach a conclusion, 76% of women who ate meat suffered from painful periods, compared to 20% of vegetarians. Fish intake did not seem to have an effect on dysmenorrhoea, even though you'd think the anti-inflammatory fatty acids counteract those in red meat.

Why can red meat cause menstrual problems? A study that showed double the risk of endometriosis with higher red meat consumption found that out of all saturated fats, only palmitic acid was linked with endometriosis. Palmitic acid is present in animal products. Yet more of the downsides to red meat may come from how it is commonly cooked, such as barbecuing (see High-AGE Foods below).

The effect of red meat may be from more than just its total fat and palmitic acid content, so only eating low-fat cuts would not help. It may be in fact due to haeme iron, the type found in animal products. Red meat contains the highest levels of haeme iron, which is what makes it red and is why conventional nutritional advice says young women should eat it. Some brands of vegetarian burgers now contain leghaemoglobin, a type of haeme naturally found in soybean roots, but we don't know the long-term effects of regularly eating it. What we do know is that haeme iron from meat has been found to trigger oxidative stress and DNA damage. This could be why even consuming red meat two to four times per week is associated with a modest increase in endometriosis risk. Although it isn't as much as eating red meat every day, this means a lot more for you if you're genetically predisposed to immune or reproductive issues. On top of this, too much haeme iron can contribute to diabetes, so it may be implicated in PCOS. Always consider: what is your family history like, and among those related to you by blood, who is the healthiest?

Dairy

Like red meat, dairy is also high in arachidonic acid; so many women must limit or remove it from their diets. However, it also provides protein, calcium, and in the case of fermented dairy foods, anti-inflammatory probiotics, so it really depends on the individual. A few months after I stopped eating both gluten and dairy, I gained a tolerance to dairy foods, starting with goat's milk yoghurt.

Dairy can be inflammatory through the presence of A1 beta-casein, a protein found in most European breeds of cattle. It's not just about lactose intolerance. A1 casein releases an often nasty substance that activates opioid receptors throughout the body. A2 casein can produce it too, but at much lower levels. What does this mean? When opioid receptors are activated in the digestive system, it slows transit time, which can lead to constipation. Constipation is not only uncomfortable, but may also increase toxin reabsorption and disrupt gut bacteria population balance.

Additionally, this "opioid" produced from A1 casein increases inflammation and attracts immune cells in a manner similar to infection. A small Australian study found higher levels of inflammation, and therefore pain and bloating, when volunteers drank A1 milk compared to A2 milk. However, they did drink 750mL of A1 milk every day, which is often too much even for people who'd normally consider themselves tolerant to dairy foods.

One reason why A1 casein is inflammatory is because it affects our ability to protect ourselves. The opioid released by the digestion of A1 casein impairs production of glutathione, a powerful antioxidant made by our bodies. When volunteers drank A2-only milk, their levels of glutathione were much higher. There was nothing in the way of their bodies using the amino acids in milk to produce glutathione. As the "master antioxidant", glutathione plays a key role in fighting inflammation by preventing and resolving tissue damage. It is tragically ironic that we are told to drink cow's milk in order to strengthen our bones, but glutathione depletion actually *weakens them*. No thanks.

Although A2 casein produces a much weaker opioid-like substance than A1, it hasn't been shown to cause harmful effects (you may react negatively, however; it depends on sensitivity). Goat's milk can be a less inflammatory alternative to dairy products from cows. In one study, the A1 casein content of goat milk was only 3.9%, almost one-tenth that of cow's milk (33.7%). It also has more short- and medium-chain fats, which are more easily digestible. My mother's cousin had terrible eczema as a child, aggravated by cow's milk, and her parents' successful solution was to keep a goat so she would have safe milk. Everyone reacts differently to dairy foods, but I recommend switching to either A2-only milks or plant-based alternatives.

However, dairy foods may in fact reduce the risk of PMS in some women. One study found that dairy intake was linked to a lower rate of PMS symptoms. However, milk and ice cream were eaten less often than yoghurt, cheese and *doogh*, a salty but refreshing Iranian drink. These are fermented and so are likely to contain anti-inflammatory probiotics such as the *Lactobacillus* species, or encourage their growth. Similar patterns of symptom reduction have also been found when taking calcium supplements.

It is important to remember that dairy products are traditional foods in Iran. If your heritage comes from regions where they were not consumed until Western colonisation, it's best for you to eat other foods that encourage *Lactobacillus spp.* growth and maintenance, such as lacto-fermented vegetables. Many, sometimes all, people of ethnic groups from North and South America, Australia, the Pacific Islands, East Asia and much of Africa do not retain tolerance to milk past early childhood.

Wheat and Gluten

I know it sounds cliched, but yes, if you have inflammatory issues then you should try going gluten-free for at least three months. This played a role in my own healing – including that of my nervous system! I thought my issues with balance, coordination and focus were from mercury fillings, but no! Coeliac disease (CD), where you absolutely cannot eat gluten, affects around 1% of Western Europeans and features a severe gastrointestinal reaction, including a flattened out intestinal lining. However, there are many more people who do not have the relevant intestinal damage or genetics for CD, but do react negatively to gluten. Some people just have the inflammatory response and the genes linked with a higher risk of CD; their needs are no less valid.

Although it isn't as strong as in patients with CD, the same inflammatory response to gluten has been found in all volunteers by multiple studies. Gliadins, which are parts of gluten, cause leaky gut in both coeliac and many non-coeliac people; it's just worse in CD. They release a protein called zonulin, which compromises the integrity of the proteins meant to keep the cells of our intestinal lining tightly knit together. Increased permeability is linked to inflammatory and autoimmune diseases, from asthma to multiple sclerosis (MS).

Wheat, barley and rye, as well as the gluten-free grains corn and rice, also contain lectins, which are antinutrients that can sometimes be toxic. The most studied is WGA, known to cause inflammation and leaky gut. People with coeliac disease have higher antibodies to WGA in their blood, meaning that it may work together with gluten to cause more damage than lectins alone. Most people are able to tolerate corn and rice. The presence of gluten and lectins together may be why many studies have found that switching to more nutritious wholegrains from refined products may aid weight loss, but won't directly reduce inflammation. On the other hand, a Paleo diet can lower some measures of inflammation, as it is grain-free. Remember that everyone is different, so you may not need to stop eating all grains. Soaking, sprouting, long cooking times and fermentation all help to reduce or remove lectins.

There has also been research specifically on how gluten can negatively affect menstruation, in particular endometriosis. A study of around 200 women found that after one year of a gluten-free diet, 156 (75%) experienced significant improvement in their symptoms. No one got worse, either. Everyone reported a considerable improvement in mental health, social and physical functioning, general health perception and vitality. This may be relevant to women who don't have endometriosis, but still have difficult periods as I once did.

Endometriosis isn't the only situation where restricting gluten improves mental health. A study of 22 people with IBS on gluten-free diets involved them taking turns on three food challenges: gluten, whey (milk protein) and a placebo. Eating gluten caused a small but significant increase in depression scores. This translates to going from a "neutral depressive" to "mild depressive" mood over the three days where they ate the protein. One person showed dramatic increases in depression and cortisol levels after consuming whey, however, which illustrates how everyone is different.

If you suffer from menstrual migraines, you could benefit from a gluten-free diet, too. In a relatively early study (2001), ten patients with gluten sensitivity, abnormal MRI scans, headaches and degrees of ataxia were instructed to avoid the offending protein. All nine who followed these instructions improved: seven no longer had headaches, and two significantly improved. The last patient didn't even try the diet. I don't know why; I can't stand losing my balance after eating gluten, and serious headaches inflict hell on patients' everyday life. In those who went back to eating gluten (again, why?), their brain abnormalities got worse. Keeping a gluten-free diet may be hard for some, but if it dramatically improves your health and allows you to live a normal life, it's worthwhile. If someone judges you or treats you like an inconvenience for having special dietary requirements, they are not your friend.

If you suspect an intolerance or allergy to gluten, dairy or something else, see a professional for one-on-one support. They will help you find the right elimination diet and additional testing if necessary. If you have already cut out a potentially offending food, they can help to confirm the problem and provide dietary advice to help prevent deficiencies. Some people who are intolerant to "normal" wheat products can have sourdough bread, others can eat gluten-containing grains that are grown in certain countries or with little to no glyphosate.

Alcohol

It may sometimes feel like an antisocial decision, but limiting alcohol consumption to special occasions can go a long way in keeping inflammation under control. It's one of my own triggers for pain, so I aim to avoid regular use. Research shows that alcohol only mildly increases the risk of PMS and PMDD, which becomes more significant with starting at a young age or long-term consumption. However, it has several negative health effects which increase inflammation.

Infla-Menses

Alcohol, especially when you drink heavily, can increase or trigger leaky gut, where the gut wall becomes too permeable and things other than nutrients are able to cross the barrier and enter the bloodstream (more on that later). This is partly caused by depletion of nutrients such as zinc. Avoiding alcohol for at least two weeks after, say, a holiday where you've been partying almost every night, is necessary for the wall to be repaired. It may take even longer if you've been drinking for a long time. Exposure to alcohol impairs the intestinal stem cells that make the fast-acting repair and maintenance of our gut walls possible. To make things worse, alcohol also impairs our normal detoxification abilities, so toxins and cellular garbage may accumulate to some degree and cause more trouble. Both acute and chronic exposure to alcohol affects the liver's natural regeneration processes too.

Why is alcohol so damaging? First, it increases oxidative stress and depletes our antioxidant reserves. In a small study where six men consumed alcohol, it reduced the level of carotenoids in their skin and made them more vulnerable to sunburn. Carotenoids are a broad class of antioxidants found in fruits and vegetables, including beta-carotene, which makes carrots orange, and lycopene, found in tomatoes. Drinking orange juice with the alcohol neutralised this effect, however, but it means you don't get a net benefit.

As we know, oxidative stress damages cells and tissues, and if you keep pouring on the cause of this damage, repair won't happen. Another toxic effect of alcohol that adds to this problem is depletion of NAD+, a modified form of vitamin B3 that we need to produce cellular energy, and therefore *definitely* need for tissue regeneration.

If you suspect that alcohol is making your menstrual problems worse, I recommend that you include how much you drink in a food diary so you can compare it to your symptoms. Even if it seems to have no effect, keeping within the Australian government's guidelines of no more than two standard drinks per night for women will help protect your health in the long run.

High-AGE Foods

Foods high in advanced glycation end-products (AGEs) include both sugary and fried foods, as well as those cooked at very high temperatures. Yes, an essential part of an anti-inflammatory diet is looking at how food is cooked, and the food combinations that you use, not just what you eat.

A special report in the August 2015 issue of *Life Extension* magazine, covering 20 pages and around 120 scientific references, aimed to inform the world about what happens when we eat too many foods cooked at high temperatures. As early as 2003, the author described a study showing that these foods speed aging by glycation of our body's tissues. Glycation is a process where sugars become tangled in our cells' and tissues' protein and fat components, which not only impairs structure and function, but also causes inflammation.

Faster aging and devastating disease may come later, but problems like period pain and PMS are often the early warning signs that we are on the wrong track – they aren't out to ruin your day, so much as they are out to help you. If you need to lose weight in order to improve your health,

Infla-Menses

reducing glycation by eating foods cooked at a lower temperature has led to more weight loss among diabetic patients than the same diet prepared at higher temperatures. They also achieved better blood glucose control.

Different foods have different levels of glycation products, and the same food can vary depending on how it's cooked. For example, steamed chicken has an average of 952 kilounits of AGEs per serving (low-AGE), but fast food nuggets have around 7,764kU in each serving (high-AGE). Homemade potato chips (French fries) have around 694kU, but fast food versions can have 1,522kU. A roasted sweet potato can contain as little as 72kU, making them one of the lowest-AGE cooked foods. You don't have to completely give up fried foods, though. I enjoy homemade bhajis – fried onion and chickpea flour fritters – but I only cook them until they are a light golden brown in a relatively small amount of coconut oil (as opposed to huge deep fryers you see used in shops).

If you enjoy toast, there's no shame in fitting the millennial stereotype of smashed avocado: a serving of avocado contains only 473kU, as opposed to 1100-1300kU for butter. My generation also gets a bit of attention for the rising popularity of vegetarian diets, and once again, it's not a bad thing. When veggie burgers were tested, they measured at up to 375kU, but a Big Mac came out as 7,800kU! In general, fruit, vegetables, wholegrains, beans, legumes and yoghurt are low-AGE, and raw nuts are better than roasted ones. Fried, roasted, grilled or broiled meats are typically the worst offenders, with bacon close to the top at just over eleven thousand kU. The more something is blackened or fried to a crisp, the more glycation products it is likely to contain.

It is best to limit meat, whether you are mostly vegetarian, pescatarian or flexitarian (where at least 75% of meat is replaced by vegetarian alternatives, or no more than five servings of meat per week). If you must eat red meat, no more than twice per month is best, preferably in a stew or curry. And remember to limit your intake of added sugar, unless sugar is absolutely necessary for a sporting event to prevent the depletion of your energy stores. High blood sugar can create internal glycation reactions that lead to serious tissue damage when it goes unabsorbed. This is why people with diabetes often suffer from nerve, blood vessel and kidney deterioration.

AGEs also trigger inflammation by making the proteins they attach to look different. It causes immune cells to form antibodies against them, as they may well be a bacterium or virus. When they attach to their receptor (appropriately named RAGE), yet more inflammation is produced; the damage to blood vessels doesn't help either. On the other hand, reducing HbA1c by 1%, or 11mmol/mol, cuts the risk of diabetes complications by 25%. Cataracts are reduced by 19%, heart failure by 16%, and amputation (or worse, death!) by 43%. It doesn't sound like much, but the effects are amazing.

There are also ways to protect against glycation products and other toxins formed by over-cooking with food. Two of the most protective nutrients are chlorophyllin, found in green vegetables, and indole-3-carbinol (I3C), found in cruciferous vegetables such as broccoli, cabbage and cauliflower. A study on chlorophyllin found that, in the dosage amount used, it can reduce the DNA-damaging effects of fried pork, coal dust and diesel emissions by over 90%! It mainly works on heterocyclic amines. These are also produced by cooking at high temperatures and another source of inflammation. As for I3C, it may cut the rate of DNA damage by up to 95% in several organs, including by a rate of up to 81% in the immune cells, and 72% in the liver. With leafy green and cruciferous vegetables, you can (occasionally) have your barbecue and eat it too.

Other nutrients that can reduce glycation are CoQ10 (150-200mg/day), magnesium (250mg/day), zinc (correct any deficiency), and vitamin D. A study on high doses of vitamin D also found that it increased antioxidant status. Finally, acidic marinades, such as those containing lemon juice or vinegar, are commonly seen in Asian and Mediterranean cuisines, and can limit glycation during cooking.

Sugar

When I was studying to become a naturopath, the nutrition world became aware that it is added and refined sugar, not fat, that contributes to obesity and chronic diseases. Why did we think that added sugar was harmless for so long? From the 1940s until recently, the sugar industry paid scientists to reach the conclusion that added sugar was safe and even healthy. This insanity went so far that in the 1980s, the Life Extension Foundation had to counteract statements by a top university professor that people should have soft drinks between meals! Now, we know how damaging it really is.

It's okay if I'm at a healthy weight, right? Actually, a study on healthy young men demonstrated that added sugar increases inflammation even when it doesn't make you gain weight. All 29 took turns following six dietary interventions for three weeks at a time: sugary drinks with a total of 40g fructose/day; 40g glucose/day; 80g fructose/day; 80g glucose/day; 80g sucrose/day and dietary advice on reducing fructose consumption. High fructose and high sucrose were the worst, more than doubling inflammation (measured as hs-CRP) from 205ng/mL to 430 and 422ng/mL respectively. The other sugary drinks weren't that much better, increasing hs-CRP to 374-394ng/mL, and the low-fructose intervention didn't totally reverse the rise in inflammation over three weeks. Fructose also significantly increased waist-to-hip ratio and body fat percentage, even though weight wasn't really affected. Added fructose (not from whole fruits) raises body fat, blood levels of fat and uric acid, leading to oxidative stress, inflammation and insulin resistance.

Population studies show that added sugar is not your friend when it comes to menstruation either. In a study of Spanish university students, the risk of dysmenorrhoea in the women who reported drinking cola soft drinks was double that of those who didn't have them. This reflected the results of another on female students in Ethiopia, where the sugary drinks again contributed to period pain. Before the results were adjusted, consumption of simple sugars and a lower fruit intake (less than three pieces per day) were also linked with a higher rate of dysmenorrhoea.

Sugary drinks can be yet another culprit in depression. In a review of 10 studies with a total of 365,289 participants, those in the highest range of sugary drink consumption had a 31% greater risk of depression compared to the lowest. The equivalent of two cans of soft drink every day was linked to a 5% higher rate of the illness, while the equivalent of three was associated with a 25% greater prevalence.

If you're struggling to keep your blood sugar and glycation levels in the healthy range, there are several supplements that may help. Zinc picolinate (a bioavailable form) may help insulin sensitivity, so if your zinc levels are below 100, supplementation could be indicated. Magnesium deficiency also causes poor glucose control and glycation; a red blood cell level of under 5.2 calls for about 500mg of magnesium glycinate. Chromium picolinate helps glucose to enter cells; it is a trace mineral, so supplement carefully with one-on-one support. Berberine, from herbal medicines such as goldenseal, also helps with blood sugar control, as does cinnamon. Cinnamon is easily accessible, and you only need one quarter of a teaspoon each day.

What about Soy?

Soy is one of the most controversial foods in the modern world, with many people either firmly for or against it. But what is the truth – should we avoid all soy; could it be used as a meat substitute all the time; or are moderate intakes of certain types of soy foods best?

First, let's look at why soy is often promoted as healthy. Its high protein content and versatility means that vegetarians and vegans do not need to fear protein deficiency or missing out on burgers. Per 100g, they have more protein than other plant sources such as chickpeas, lentils and peanuts. They are also rich in B vitamins, iron, zinc, calcium and fats, which are mostly polyunsaturated and help us to stay satisfied without reaching for chips or a chocolate bar. The bean's fibre content is easily fermentable by gut bacteria, so it can act as a prebiotic. Tofu can be particularly high in calcium when it is made with calcium sulphate curd. Other traditional preparations are the fermented foods tempeh, soy sauce, sufu and natto.

Besides essential nutrients, soy isoflavones may be protective against certain diseases such as breast cancer. These are known as genistein, daidzein and glycitein. Population studies have found that East Asian women have a 30% lower risk of the illness if they regularly consume soy. However, this may only apply to those who began to eat soy during childhood, the earlier the better. Isoflavones appear to permanently change cells in developing breast tissue in ways that make them less likely to become cancerous. They may also reduce mortality rates in women with triple-negative breast cancers, which do not respond to hormone therapies.

Not every woman will develop breast cancer, but every woman will go through menopause. The isoflavone genistein is able to significantly relieve hot flashes with less concern over side effects than conventional HRT. Soy intake can halve their severity, compared to a 75% reduction seen with estrogen replacement therapy. On the other hand, a mixture of the three can improve bone calcium levels in post-menopausal women.

What about menstrual problems, such as endometriosis? A Japanese study on over 130 women with the disease found that higher urinary levels of genistein and daidzein were linked with a lower risk of advanced endometriosis. Women in the top 25% for daidzein levels had a 71% lower risk, while those in the top 25% for genistein had a 79% lower risk of advanced disease. Overall, higher levels of isoflavones were associated with reduced severity. There was no link between them and early-stage endometriosis. Much of this effect was because of their oestrogen receptor-modulating properties. In Japan, a woman's soy intake is more likely to feature traditional fermented foods than unfermented processed products.

As for the argument against soy, many benefits of soy consumption may simply be misplaced attribution or only relevant in certain situations. It is often eaten as a replacement for meat or dairy, "protecting" us against cardiovascular disease by standing in for potentially inflammatory foods. Compared to Western meat and dairy alternatives, traditional fermented foods also contain more readily absorbed forms of isoflavones. Additionally, their positive effects seem to be determined by our intestinal microbiome's ability to produce equol from isoflavones. The bacteria responsible for this are supported by a diet low in saturated fats and high in total carbohydrates; antibiotic use reduces equol levels.

We know that soy isoflavones aren't protective against breast cancer if consumption begins in adulthood, and an overall healthy diet is paramount, but what about any harms? Research has found that soy flavonoids may inhibit thyroid function, at least alongside low iodine intake. Another study on Adventist women showed a lower probability of becoming a mother with higher isoflavone intakes. The strongest relationship was found among women who reported difficulty in falling pregnant. Marriage and education level were controlled for, making it less likely that the women were childfree by choice. Researchers have documented at least two cases of male feminisation too, but these were in men consuming an unusually high quantity of soy.

Another issue with soy is its high level of lectins. Excessive lectin intake can disrupt nutrient absorption, raise inflammation, impact serotonin signaling and cause fatigue. They do this by binding to the intestinal wall and causing leaky gut syndrome. To make things worse, lectins can damage cells by acting like insulin and allowing glucose to flood in. Existing health problems such as autoimmune diseases can trigger or worsen lectin sensitivity, so not everyone is seriously affected. Besides avoidance, you can limit lectin exposure by only consuming fermented soy foods and thorough cooking.

The greatest health concern when it comes to soy intake is the presence of glyphosate. Non-organic soy is commonly genetically modified to be "Roundup Ready", so it can tolerate large amounts of glyphosate. I will discuss this herbicide later on. Organic soy is higher in protein and zinc, while containing lower levels of omega-6 fatty acids. Therefore, the best soy foods are organic, fermented and made by traditional methods instead of modern over-processing. If you have a thyroid condition or are having trouble conceiving, seek professional advice or simply consume other nutrient-dense plant foods.

Lifestyle and Environmental Factors

Chronic Infections

Chronic infections, including Lyme disease; viruses, such as *Herpes simplex*, moulds like *Aspergillus* or *Penicillium*, and oral bacteria such as *P. gingivalis* can all cause or worsen inflammation. Then, on the other hand, long-term antibiotic exposure is also inflammatory, so it is important to resolve these infections as soon as possible. I say exposure because meat and other animal foods from industrial agriculture operations contain antibiotics. What's cruel for the planet and animal life is cruel for us. I recommend trying to source eggs and dairy from friends or small businesses; local social media groups may help.

Why are they so difficult to treat, compared to, say, a cold? One of my own articles, *Can't Beat Chronic Infections? Try Busting Biofilms*, published in Honey Colony in 2018, discusses how chronic infections can cause "non-infectious" long-term health problems, why they are so stubborn and how to kick them out of your life.

Chronic infections with biofilm involvement are often unresponsive to antibiotics alone. Biofilms are slimy combinations of protein, fats and carbohydrates that keep the immune system and antimicrobials from getting rid of the pathogens hiding underneath. An example of how stubborn they are is Lyme disease, where patients often struggle for years to find the best treatment. Biofilms also contribute to chronic inflammatory illness by overstimulating the immune system. The illnesses they cause include Crohn's disease, ulcerative colitis, arthritis, fibromyalgia and chronic fatigue syndrome. These seem to be common in young women.

When they produce proteins that look similar to our own for the biofilms, the immune system can get confused and start to attack both.

So what can we do to get rid of them? Certain enzymes, in particular serrapeptase, may help to break up biofilms. This one has been shown to interfere with *S. aureus* biofilm formation. Some formulations have other enzymes, such as amylase for the carbohydrate component, protease for proteins and cellulase for cellulose. Many of these are found in digestive enzyme supplements, but it's best to enlist professional help so you can get something specific for chronic infections. You'd have suffered enough to waste more time on a basic digestion blend. A good one will have the right combination to fight the different biofilm formations produced by different pathogens.

A woman I interviewed for the Honey Colony article, "Julia", took 23 years to fully recover from chronic infections. Epstein-Barr virus and toxoplasmosis (from cat faeces) left her with chronic fatigue syndrome, and so an integrative doctor advised her to avoid wheat and dairy, while putting her on vitamin C, Chinese herbs and other supplements. She returned to study, but couldn't exercise and was always tired after 5:00pm. Homeopathic GABA, magnesium and omega-3 fats helped her recover more normalcy and work full-time. Years later, new symptoms appeared, and she was diagnosed with *Blastocystis colitis*, other parasites, Rickettsia and the "Australian version of Lyme disease". Then, her integrative doctor put her on doxycycline for 11 months, but her treatment felt like it was on hold until a naturopath recommended Interfase Plus. At the time of writing, she hadn't needed antibiotics for eight months, hadn't needed a daytime nap for one month and was even regaining energy at night. However, she still needed supplementation and to watch her diet. Interfase Plus contains enzymes and EDTA, a binder that helps to detach bacteria. Modified citrus pectin is another binder that disrupts biofilms, but won't deplete you of essential minerals like EDTA does. Ensure that you supplement with beneficial minerals, such as calcium, magnesium, iron and zinc, if you need a blend that contains EDTA.

Some probiotic species may also break up biofilms. *Lactobacillus acidophilus*, *L. casei* and *L. rhamnosus* have been found to reduce cell counts in *Candida* biofilms by 25-61%, depending on the probiotic species and stage of biofilm development. In this case, *L. rhamnosus* only inhibited early-stage biofilms. They did not behave like antibiotics, but interrupted Candida cells' communication and ability to colonise surfaces. *L. acidophilus* can reduce mature *S. aureus* biofilms by 83%, but this drops to 15% for early-stage biofilms. Probiotics can also help to maintain healthy intestinal flora and reduce the side effects of antibiotics, so don't wait to finish your course of pharmaceutical or herbal antimicrobials.

Other natural remedies for biofilms include N-acetyl cysteine. At least in combination with antibiotics, it can thin out mucus in biofilms, eliminate mature biofilms and kill off the infection. Additionally, compounds in garlic, particularly allicin and ajoene, can disrupt biofilm formation in some bacteria and *Candida albicans*, as well as interrupt bacterial communication. Finally, ozone therapy may help too. A study of biofilms taken from children with cystic fibrosis found that 30 seconds of exposure to ozonated water, or 40 minutes of exposure to ozone gas, started to reduce the bacterial counts. You would most likely need a combination of therapies, so please consult a professional instead of trying to fight chronic infections on your own.

Toxic Mould

Just because you can't see it, doesn't mean it can't hurt you. Water damage in your home can invite toxic species of mould to grow, which produce allergens and irritants. Even though so many patients with illnesses caused by toxic mould started out healthy and high-achieving, the predominant belief was that they were imagining it. Fortunately, the truth is coming out.

Around 1500 Australians have already been diagnosed with Chronic Inflammatory Response Syndrome (CIRS), caused by a build-up of toxins that mould species produce. A syndrome is a condition defined by a pattern of signs and symptoms that may not be the same for everyone. One of the most publicised cases is that of MP Lucy Wicks. A tree crashed through her house, and the resulting mould growth seriously disrupted the balance of her immune system. Then sensitised to mould, certain places would "turn her brain to mush", making her lose her place in conversations. She even developed asthma and pneumonia several times. To start healing, she had to move.

Of course, you don't have to develop asthma, pneumonia or short-term memory problems to have a mould-related illness. The diverse ways that these toxins affect the body mean that you could be diagnosed with chronic fatigue, dermatitis, a neurological disorder or something else entirely.

Infla-Menses

When I wrote an article on toxic mould for an integrative clinic, their head naturopath Reine DuBois said to me that "All chronic health conditions could be the result of mould, if you are part of the 25% of the population that carry the HLA genotype susceptibility". HLA gene variations affect the immune system's vulnerability to autoimmune and hypersensitive states. In Lucy Wicks' case, her mother was also mould-sensitive, so she may have had the "right" gene variation to trigger this syndrome.

How do we solve this problem? First, prevent mould growth with proper moisture control. Ensure that all rooms are sufficiently ventilated, and leave the fan on or window open for roughly 30 minutes in your bathroom after showering. Repair all leaky plumbing or spots in your walls or roof, even if you rarely venture into that room. Dry all water-damaged areas after severe weather as soon as possible (preferably within 24 hours). Cleaning off mould requires water and detergent, but you still need to let it completely dry. Unfortunately, you would probably have to replace any absorbent damaged material such as carpet.

Some patients still suffer from toxic mould-related illness long after they have moved, or their homes are cleaned and restored. Mould species such as *Aspergillus* and *Penicillium* can infect the nasal and sinus cavities, and continue to secrete toxins that can be detected throughout the body. As seen in other chronic infections, they use a biofilm to protect themselves from the immune system. Treatment is therefore similar to what I have written above for other biofilm-associated infections, and you need to see a professional one-on-one for personalised intervention.

Although the exact list of symptoms varies by person, if you are starting to become concerned that your health problems are caused by toxic mould, the Biotoxin Cluster Questionnaire may point you in the right direction. Mould-related illness is likely if you score more than eight, and a "yes" to any symptom in each cluster is a "yes" overall.

1.	Fatigue	Yes/No
2.	Weakness, difficulty learning new information, headache, light sensitivity and/or muscle aches/pains	Yes/No
3.	Poor memory and/or difficulty finding words	Yes/No
4.	Poor concentration	Yes/No
5.	Cramps, joint pain and/or morning stiffness	Yes/No
6.	Burning, numbness and/or tingling in hands and feet	Yes/No
7.	Shortness of breath and/or sinus congestion	Yes/No
8.	Cough, excessive thirst and/or confusion	Yes/No
9.	Urinary frequency, varying appetite and/or difficulty regulating body temp	Yes/No
10.	Red eyes, blurred vision, sweats, mood swings and/or ice-pick pain	Yes/No
11.	Abdominal pain, diarrhoea and/or numbness	Yes/No
12.	Tearing, metallic taste in mouth and/or disorientation	Yes/No
13.	Static shocks and/or vertigo	Yes/No

Dysbiosis and Leaky Gut

New research is uncovering exactly how powerful the intestinal microbiome is when it comes to living longer and healthier. While it was once overlooked, we are gaining a better understanding of how dysbiosis leads to a range of inflammatory, neurological and age-related diseases. For example, constipation can appear as early as 15 years before motor impairment in neurological disorders. This is because one role of a healthy microbiome is to help maintain the blood-brain barrier (BBB), so toxins that could damage the brain stay out.

Aging (or inflammaging) is related to a declining diversity and population of anti-inflammatory species. One study revealed that 53% of the microbiome in people over 65 belonged to the *Bacterioidetes* phyla (*Firmicutes* was also dominant), compared to 8-27% in younger adults. Also, people 105 and over are likely to have species from the *Ruminococcaceae*, *Lachnospiraceae* and *Bacteroidaceae* families. These usually fall in numbers with age, but help us to live longer if they stick around. They also help *Akkermansia*, *Bifidobacterium*, already in many probiotics; and *Christenellaceae*, which is linked with improved kidney function. *Akkermansia* species are other producers of anti-inflammatory short-chain fatty acids. Overall, there is a pattern of greater diversity, anti-inflammatory species, and some similarities to younger people in centenarians. As these findings are so new, we still need to learn about which foods encourage their presence and how to best formulate probiotics with them, but let's keep their names in mind for now so we know what to look for later.

Dysbiosis also causes leaky gut, where the wall becomes too permeable and things that shouldn't be in the bloodstream can enter. Gluten sensitivity, pesticides, sugary foods (added, not fruit in moderation), alcohol, processed food, preservatives, stress, yeast and drugs such as aspirin or acetaminophen are other causes. When the gut wall is "leaky", inflammatory immune chemicals can enter the bloodstream and travel to other organs, such as the uterus and even the brain. A leaky gut allows intestinal bacteria to enter out-of-bounds areas such as the bloodstream and lymphatic system too. This triggers a necessary inflammatory response in order to remove them, as even the friendly species seen in probiotics have their right and wrong places to be. They do help our immune system stay in balance, as well as aid digestion, but must stay in the digestive tract where they belong.

Sometimes, undigested proteins, bacteria, yeast and fragments of these can resemble our own tissues and confuse our immune system. Then, you get chronic inflammation and maybe even autoimmune disease. Although she did not have Alzheimer's disease, Dr Dale Bredesen details the case of a young woman with lupus, including arthritis, who learnt that she had leaky gut and food sensitivities. Her symptoms disappeared with nutritional medicine and hormone rebalancing treatment, but they came back whenever she ate gluten. The lesson is: stay on your treatment plan. Your body has an amazing memory when it comes to identifying threats, so don't undo months of healing for the sake of fitting in.

Infla-Menses

Dysbiosis has been directly linked with menstrual problems too. Endometriosis may be associated with a lower intestinal population of *Lactobacillus spp.* and a higher proportion of gram-negative bacteria, as well as *Candida*. There can also be more intestinal inflammation. It is most likely a cycle of cause and effect, not just intestinal inflammation causing endometriosis or the other way around.

Additionally, women with PCOS often have a lower level of diversity in their intestinal flora. A study of 73 women with PCOS, 42 with polycystic ovaries who did not fit the symptomatic criteria, and 48 healthy women found that less diversity was related to more severe symptoms. Those with cysts but not PCOS had an intermediate level of diversity.

Some species of bacteria were higher in women with PCOS, including those that can contribute to leaky gut and dysbiosis, as well as others found at higher levels in obese or diabetic people. The four groups (taxa, for biology enthusiasts) present at lower populations all produce SCFAs, which are anti-inflammatory and aid immunity. One SCFA, butyrate, even reduces the power of pathogenic bacteria. Decreased levels of some of these species are linked with Crohn's disease and ulcerative colitis. While the path of causation is unclear in this study – do hormone imbalances cause dysbiosis, or does dysbiosis cause hormonal issues? – there would still be an inflammatory aspect of PCOS. Some of these species may also help to metabolise hormones.

EMF Exposure

Communication technologies such as mobile phones have dramatically improved our access to information and ability to stay in contact with friends, regardless of where you are in the world. However, we can have too much of a good thing because they are a source of electromagnetic frequency (EMF) radiation.

In a review of 100 studies, 93 demonstrated that EMF radiation increases oxidative stress. This is partly because it is possible to become allergic to EMF, with mast cells (a type of immune cell involved in allergies) increasing in areas of the body exposed to the radiation. The immune cells respond as if the EMF were a disease-causing microbe, triggering the inflammatory response to remove it. Oxidative stress caused by EMF radiation can damage any part of the cell or tissue, such as the DNA or mitochondria (the energy-producing, miniature "organs" of the cell). Once again, an inflammatory response would be triggered if the cell is killed off, in order to mop up the damage. As oxidative stress and inflammation can turn into a nasty cycle, do not keep your mobile phone in your pockets either (i.e. close to your uterus), just as you wouldn't in your bra.

We are not informed by conventional sources about the large volume of research warning against constant EMF exposure. On the other hand, if a pharmaceutical drug had even half the number of studies demonstrating that it was effective, it would be approved and widely seen as evidence-based medicine. So why is there never enough evidence against too much EMF radiation?

Infla-Menses

Sometimes, results depend on design. When studies on EMF safety were analysed, researchers found that only mobile phone use for over ten years was associated with significant harmful effects, so it's never too early or too late to moderate your exposure. Industry-funded research does not show significant damage to our health, for obvious reasons, but higher-quality studies generally show stronger effects.

Of course, moderation is always best, and seek help if you have an addiction to online activities such as social media use or video games. Don't store your phone in your bra or pocket; keep it in your bag, locker or on a table when you aren't using it. When you do use a computer or phone, I recommend a headset or the speaker. I usually sit my phone on the table or armrest instead of holding it too. If you have a Wi-Fi system in your house, please turn it off when it is not in use! You don't need it on overnight; the same goes for your phone (turn Flight Mode on if you need the alarm). I also do not recommend wearable technology. Reliance on activity tracker apps and being totally dependent on your phone creates issues for privacy too – something essential for your personal freedom, but inconvenient to corporations. So what if you have nothing to hide? You have nothing to owe either; you were meant to be wild and free, not tagged and tracked!

Obesity

Obesity is nothing trivial – it is regarded as the epidemic of the 21st century. Several hundred million people around the world are obese, and many more are overweight. This threatens to stop the continuous gains seen in life expectancy, through a wide range of diseases at least partly caused by inflammation. You see, fat cells are not just for storage, but help to regulate hormone balance and the immune system. They don't cause any harm in people with a normal proportion of body fat, but in obesity their functions become dysregulated, and the immune cells that work with them produce too many inflammatory chemicals. "Too many" can mean up to ten times the normal level! Abdominal fat, i.e. that lying around the organs, has the highest production rate of these inflammatory substances.

Inflammation also contributes to weight gain itself, with more inflammatory markers associated with a larger future increase in body weight. This was adjusted for physical activity, alcohol, smoking, insulin resistance, baseline weight, and height, to make sure that it was the most likely cause. The harmful cycle that this creates is one more reason why it can be so hard to lose excess weight.

An unhealthy weight will also put you at greater risk for menstrual issues like period pain now; it's not just a question of chronic disease and a shorter lifespan later. A 13-year study of almost ten thousand women found that starting off as underweight or obese was linked with a higher risk of period pain. If they were underweight, their risk was 34% higher; if they were obese, then they were 22% more likely to have it. Women who stayed underweight or obese still had a 33% greater risk, but obese women who lost weight were no more likely to experience period pain than those who were always of a normal weight. This is most likely caused by a combination of both inflammatory and hormonal factors.

Infla-Menses

The first step in fighting obesity is to see a healthcare professional who has studied holistic nutrition, such as a naturopath or Ayurvedic practitioner. The right diet for you will be different to the next person's. For example, one of my cousins can only remain at her optimal weight (and stay in good health) as long as she's on the low-carb, high/healthy fat (LCHF) diet, but others find great success with the Mediterranean diet. It is also essential to find physical activity that you enjoy, and find a gym or personal trainer if you need to deliberately work out in order to reach your goals.

Don't worry if being overweight or obese runs in your family, either. The same genes can be expressed in an entirely different way depending on diet, and we can see this in the story of Arizona's Pima Indians. They were fit and lean while living on their traditional foods until roughly 1890, but now have the highest obesity rate in the USA. This is because the government overtook their water supply and forced them to rely on "modern foods" such as white flour, sugar and junk foods when they could no longer grow their own crops. However, a group of Pimas that splintered off and migrated to Mexico kept their traditional diet and lean physiques.

Even certain types of exercise can tone down the effects of obesity-related genes. For this study, a grand total of 18,424 Chinese adults had their genetic risk scores for five obesity measures compared to their level of physical activity. These measures were BMI, waist circumference, hip circumference, waist-to-hip ratio and body fat percentage. Out of 18 types of self-reported regular exercise, six positively affected genetic effects on at least one obesity measure. Regular jogging came out on top, acting against genetic predispositions for higher BMI, hip circumference and body fat percentage. Walking, exercise walking, mountain climbing, "international standard" dancing and long yoga sessions also affected BMI. One caveat to this study is that some self-reported physical activities showing no effect, such as swimming, have very open-ended definitions. A swim could mean a dip or ten laps, while jogging or mountain climbing have certain degrees of intensity by design.

The saying "energy in, energy out" does not include everything we need to do in order to fight obesity. We must also watch out for obesogens – things that cause fat gain outside of extra energy intake. In foods, the major ones to avoid are fructose, genistein and monosodium glutamate (MSG). Fructose is the sugar found in fruits; while you shouldn't give up whole fruit, stop consuming anything with added fructose, such as high-fructose corn syrup (HFCS) containing soft drinks. Genistein comes from soy, and even though this isoflavone does have beneficial effects, avoid it if you are oestrogen-dominant or overweight. MSG is a flavour enhancer popular with Chinese restaurants, and found in many processed foods. I find that MSG not only makes foods too salty, but it can give me hand tremors and skin rashes! Environmental toxins that can contribute to obesity are discussed below.

Smoking

We now know that smoking tobacco is extremely unhealthy, with PSAs and warning labels reminding everyone that smoking now may cause cancer, cardiovascular disease or other problems later. Unfortunately, many ignore these warnings and repeat to themselves that "life is short" and "they'd rather enjoy themselves now", but did you know that smoking can cause noticeable problems, well, now?

A study of 165 young Chinese women found that exposure to cigarette smoke increased the risk of period pain from 9.7% to 13.3%. More exposure meant a greater risk, with "high" levels of smoke tripling the chance of period pain. Average daily exposures ranged from almost none to 10.3 cigarettes, so even half a pack counted as "high". This study also only counted environmental exposure – second-hand smoke – at home, and only involved women with no previous period pain. If you are genetically more vulnerable to menstrual problems or you smoke yourself, they may be even more harmful.

The Chinese research was on exposure to second-hand smoke, but what about smoking yourself? An Australian study of over 9,000 women found that the toxic habit was linked to a 41% higher risk of chronic dysmenorrhoea. Former smokers didn't have it much better with a 33% higher risk. This means that if you do smoke, don't just quit and expect all your inflammatory issues to go away. You most likely need a comprehensive treatment plan to break the cycle of chronic inflammation. Smoking can also increase the risk of PMS. One of the many studies nested in The Nurses' Health Study II followed almost 3,000 women for ten years, including 1,057 who developed PMS. Women who were smoking at the time had over twice the risk (2.1 times) of developing PMS, compared to never-smokers.

The best tobacco alternative is nothing at all, because even vaping has toxic effects. A 2018 study tested a number of different e-cigarette flavours, and not even the solution used as a vehicle was safe for cells lining the respiratory tract. Overall, a longer list of ingredients led to greater toxicity, with vanillin being a particularly nasty ingredient on inhalation. Some flavours were only slightly toxic, such as Popcorn, which dented live cell counts. Chocolate Fudge was more dangerous and obliterated over 80% of them.

The belief that vaping is safe comes from the fact that e-cigarettes do not create the toxic products of tobacco combustion, such as tar-phase chemicals. However, their use does generate by-products that cause oxidative stress (and therefore inflammation). Some flavourings also test positive for safety when ingested orally but are toxic on inhalation. In fact, a butter flavouring "generally recognised" as safe when eaten may cause scarring and blockage of the small airways!

Toxins

" The conversation has shifted from, 'Here is your destiny, get used to it!' to 'Here is your destiny, and you can do something about it" - George Church

Man-made chemical toxins, as well as the release of "natural" poisons such as heavy metals and particulate matter from fossil or wood fuels, are linked with obesity and chronic inflammatory illnesses. The rise in chronic disease is not caused by living longer, lower childhood mortality (it was about survival of the fortunate, not the fittest) or genetics, and can only be partially explained by nutrition and lifestyle.

Since World War Two, around 80,000 chemicals that our bodies just aren't made to deal with have been registered with the US government. A common saying, "the dose makes the poison", is not always relevant because toxicity has been found at extremely low doses in some cases. That saying comes from the 16th century, a time when there was a smaller range of familiar natural poisons more easily dealt with by common sense (for example, by not eating pufferfish). Its twin argument of "natural doesn't mean safe" ignores the avoidability of natural toxins, compared to the ability of man-made chemicals to migrate and persist in the environment.

Some toxins have been found to negatively affect the menstrual cycle. For example, PCBs and DDE are linked to irregular or longer cycles. Other research set out to see if PCBs and organochlorine pesticides had a relationship with irregular menstruation. These are two types of persistent organic pollutants (POPs), which stay around in the environment for years and are hard to detoxify. Different chemicals had varying effects, and sometimes the same chemical seemed to affect the menstrual cycle differently depending on the study. For example, DDT exposure may shorten the cycle, while fungicides can reduce bleeding time (the worst way to lighten your flow ever!). The effects of these were attributed to their effects on hormones.

Besides disrupting hormonal balance, pesticides and other toxins can have direct inflammatory effects. Population studies find that higher exposure to these chemicals is linked with greater levels of immune cell disruption and inflammation. For example, organophosphate pesticides are toxic to our fatty tissue (such as the brain!), cause oxidative stress and are directly inflammatory. They also overstimulate the insulin-producing cells of the pancreas and interfere with their ability to communicate. While most of these studies involve agricultural workers and their family members, we are all exposed to pesticides to some degree, and it will take a collective effort to end this by phasing out their use.

Additionally, the neurotoxic effects of mercury are at least partly caused by inflammation. In a lab study, exposing immune cells to the heavy metal led to a significant rise in inflammatory markers, including those responsible for allergic reactions. It can disrupt the blood-brain barrier too. Mercury is found in certain dental fillings and pharmaceuticals, as well as personal and home care products, fungicides, pesticides, and some species of fish. Burning coal has released mercury into the atmosphere, but some animals (including seafood staples, like tuna) accumulate it more than others. If you eat fish, remember the SMASH acronym: Salmon, Mackerel, Anchovies, Sardines and Herring; these are the safest.

Obesogens

As I wrote above, another way that these chemicals can ruin our health is by contributing to the obesity epidemic. Many toxins are stored in fat, so if you are overweight or obese, be careful when losing weight! Toxins such as endocrine-disrupting chemicals (EDCs) can also make it harder to lose unwanted weight and keep it off. These include pesticides, phthalates, dioxins, heavy metals, solvents, PCBs and flame retardants.

Two of the worst pesticides, in terms of contributing to obesity, are the EDCs atrazine and DDE (a breakdown product of DDT). These have been linked to increased BMI in children, and insulin resistance at least in rodents. Other obesogenic pesticides include the organophosphates chlorpyrifos, diazinon and parathion. If you grow your own food, please go organic; if you own a farm, research ways to go organic on a large scale or at least reduce your pesticide use (this includes herbicides, fungicides and insecticides).

Phthalates, BPA, and sometimes organotins, are obesogens we see in plastics and many other synthetic materials. BPA and phthalates have been linked to increased body weight and fat in both children and adults. Besides plastics, phthalates are found in chemical personal care products, laundry products and air fresheners. Organotins are less well-known, but can trigger stem cells to become fat instead of bone tissue; these can be found in products such as handbags and blinds. PBDEs were used in the production of mattresses as flame retardants until they were phased out from 2004 to 2013 (in the USA), while PCBs were banned from new electrical appliances in 1977. However, they continue to persist in the environment – see below for general detoxification tips. Perfluoro-octanoic acid (PFOA) is yet another persistent obesogen, used for non-stick cookware, waterproof clothing and stain repellent. Sometimes, tap water is contaminated with it, such as during a 2005 incident in West Virginia. Extra attention to detoxification is also needed if you live in an area where fine particulate matter or lead pollute the air.

Finally, oestradiol (a form of oestrogen) is a pharmaceutical obesogen. You may be on the oral contraceptive pill to prevent issues like period pain, and are reading this book to get off it, because of unwanted weight gain. I took the natural route in order to avoid this and other side effects of hormonal contraception.

So what can we do about toxins?

The first step is avoidance of your own exposure. Purchasing organic food and other products wherever possible; investing in a water filter, which cuts down on your plastic consumption; and switching to a natural mattress when it's time to change it are some ways that we can not only reduce our own chemical exposure, but also be kinder to the health of humanity and the planet. Single-use plastic bags – already banned in my corner of the world – and similar items are already on their way out in many regions too. When choosing a water filter, reverse osmosis and multi-stage cartridges (check what they are and their purpose first) are best, as long as you replenish beneficial minerals.

Don't wait for everyone else to follow in your footsteps, either; detoxification is typically an important part of healing inflammatory health complaints. One way to safely detox is by sweating, which can help remove toxins that the liver, kidneys and bloodstream have trouble with. Either exercise or a sauna can be effective. Some helpful nutrients and phytochemicals are turmeric; garlic and onions; selenium, with the richest source being Brazil nuts; B vitamins, found in sources including leafy green vegetables and wholegrains; fibre; various antioxidants and chlorella, an edible algae used as a functional food. There are also supplements such as N-acetylcysteine; MSM and lipoic acid. These work by reducing toxin absorption or reabsorption, such as with fibre; reducing damage, for example the antioxidants; or directly assisting detoxification, like garlic, Brazil nuts and chlorella. The best remedies for you depend on your individual needs.

What about glyphosate?

Infla-Menses

At the time of writing, the general population seems to be more aware of glyphosate's toxic effects than any other pesticide or herbicide ingredient. People are becoming dissatisfied with the old "bad luck" mentality and starting to ask questions if not demand action. But instead of just waiting for it to be banned, what can we do?

First of all, non-organic lentils, chickpeas, soy, oats, corn and wheat can be very high in glyphosate. It is used both as a herbicide and sprayed on as a dessicant before harvest, so it is best to choose organic versions of these foods. Totally eliminating glyphosate from the environment and food supply will take a team effort, as it is known to travel through soil and water, but there are ways to detoxify from it. Microbes of the *Acetobacter* species can fully metabolise the toxin, and these are found in certain fermented foods such as apple cider vinegar, sauerkraut, kombucha, kimchi and kefir. A study on cows exposed to glyphosate found that a combination of sauerkraut juice, activated charcoal, fulvic acid and humic acid can remove it from the body and help to relieve its toxic effects. Another on chickens also demonstrated humic acid to be effective. Fulvic and humic acid come from the soil, as part of its organic matter. It's no different to using medicinal clays as detoxification aids. Glyphosate can also be broken down by ozone therapy, but be careful if you are debilitated as it does have pro-oxidant properties.

Glyphosate impairs protein digestion and causes leaky gut, among other problems, so it is indirectly pro-inflammatory. When new diagnoses of coeliac disease, the most severe form of gluten intolerance, were compared to the use of glyphosate, numbers rose as use went up, and dropped when the amount sprayed fell. As the commercial formulations containing it can be one thousand times more dangerous than the "active ingredient" alone, its harms are underestimated when tested in isolation.

Glyphosate inhibits protein synthesis, to put it simply, in plants, bacteria and fungi. This is why everyone believed that it was safe until we learnt that our gut bacteria are necessary for life and health. Some bacteria are more vulnerable than others – pathogenic bacteria have been found in some research to be less so than *Lactobacillus* and *Bifidobacterium* species. One of the amino acids (the building blocks of protein) that glyphosate impairs production of is tryptophan, but our friendly species of bacteria need it to prevent the activity of pathogens. When they can grow unchecked, they increase zonulin and allow inflammatory chemicals, bacteria and undigested food into the bloodstream. These effects may have been why replacing red meat with soy-based vegetarian alternatives, despite its inflammatory properties, did not benefit me. The only "upside" to any of this is that the zonulin reaction is quickly reversed.

The toxic effects of glyphosate may also extend to the development of PCOS. Zonulin is higher in women with the condition, and is linked with the severity of insulin resistance and menstrual problems. Both gluten and certain bacteria (or lack thereof) can Increase zonulin, which is how glyphosate damages the gut lining. Although glyphosate is so widespread, it is "only" 5-10% of women who develop PCOS because of genetic vulnerability and the wrong combination of lifestyle factors. If it seems like genes equal destiny, we just don't have these pesticides banned long enough in enough places to create a control group.

Infla-Menses

Glyphosate may also affect you if you have emotional symptoms of PMS, PMDD, or other mental health issues. Inflammation, including that caused by leaky gut, can result in tryptophan being "stockpiled" by immune cells, creating the deficiency that may lead to serotonin depletion and therefore mental health problems like depression. Part of our tryptophan intake comes from the gut bacteria, and if this is blocked by toxins such as glyphosate, our levels of it may fall. To make things worse, tryptophan is used to make NAD+, a vitamin B3 derivative we need to produce energy and repair DNA. This is being studied as an antiaging intervention – let's not deplete it! And there's just that "little" problem of the obesity epidemic. Serotonin prevents overeating, and the obesity crisis began soon after glyphosate's introduction in the USA. Once again, harming the environment harms our health and longevity too. We are not a pest on the Earth; we are the Earth and separation is only an illusion.

Can I Still Wear Makeup?

A major source of toxic exposure for women is chemical cosmetics, which is why I recommend the use of natural alternatives. These can be anything from simple homemade recipes to high-end, certified organic brands. There are many resources out there for you to make your own natural cosmetics, including the ebook *Make Your Own Makeup From Organic Food or Minerals* from The Health Extremist.

Conventional hair dyes, however, are possibly the most toxic product you can get. If you don't want to go grey, or simply want a change of hair colour, there are safe natural alternatives out there, including henna-based tints and dyes.

Henna produces a red colour, so many dyes mix it with other plant pigments like the black/deep blue indigo. As I have very dense, dandruff-prone hair, I found that one of the best things for my hair is a conditioner with a mild henna tint. It doesn't just look good, but can be a fantastic antimicrobial and antifungal (dandruff often has fungal involvement). The phytochemical in henna responsible for its red pigment, lawsone, is also largely responsible for its antimicrobial properties. Lawsone is effective against *Candida albicans*, while experiments with henna leaf extract found "absolute toxicity" against ringworm-causing species, including *Microsporum gypseum* and *Trichophyton mentagrophytess.*

Menstrual Hygiene

What you use during your period can significantly affect your exposure to toxins too. Although I was taught to use disposable pads and tampons, I eventually switched to a reusable silicone menstrual cup (with accompanying plant-based wash) to reduce my usage of plastic. Soon after I started using the cup, I noticed that I had less inflammation, a bonus when I already loved the absence of itchy, sweaty, nappy-like pads. There is far less cotton in sanitary pads than commonly advertised; in fact, they are mostly plastic and may contain the equivalent of up to four plastic bags!

This doesn't just have harmful effects on the environment. A study published in March 2019 found that sanitary pads contain more phthalates than other common plastic products, and can be very high in volatile organic compounds (VOCs). The worst offenders contained 5,900 times more VOCs and 130 times more phthalates than the cleanest pads. They also, unlike plastic bags, spend several hours in contact with a sensitive area of the body, and are

Infla-Menses

likely to release these chemicals into the reproductive organs and bloodstream.

To avoid them and their impact on the environment, switch to a reusable menstrual cup made of medical-grade silicone or latex rubber, or washable organic cotton pads. Some have measuring markers on the inside – my cup has 7.5mL and 15mL marks – so they can be more helpful in monitoring a heavy flow too. Australian consumer group CHOICE has the guide, *How to Buy the Best Menstrual Cup For You*, which compares the Juju, Ruby, Diva Cup (my brand), MoonCup, Keeper, Lunette and Lily Cup, and outlines the pros and cons of using a cup. Cleaning and insertion can take some getting used to, but they are cheaper, more comfortable, better suited to an active lifestyle, and save roughly 250 pads each year (or an average of 11,000 over your menstruating years). *Menstrual Cup Reviews* advises on both cups and reusable pads, such as the Lunapad, which features removable inserts (meaning less laundry).

Negative Emotions

If you have menstrual problems or inflammatory disorders in general, you may notice that they get worse during stressful times. It's not just because you feel like rubbish; negative emotions do affect physical health, because everything in us is connected.

First, stress and depression are no good for immune balance. They delay wound healing, increase risk of infection, prolong infections and raise inflammation in the absence of these things. Poor sleep, a consequence of stress and depression, also raises IL-6. In one study using a stressor, NF-kB activity rose by 341% - over four times – in 10 minutes! Noradrenaline, one of the stress hormones, promotes NF-kB activation, another reason why treatment for menstrual problems often needs both inflammation and endocrine balance to be addressed.

You don't necessarily "just get used to" long-term stress either. Studies on people who do intensive unpaid caring work (e.g. for loved ones with dementia, or seriously ill children) found that the stress magnified inflammation, measured as IL-6, by four times compared to the usual level for their age, as well as oxidative stress.

Poor emotional health is not only inflammatory itself; it also influences dietary choices. Stress can throw out the normal metabolic response to even healthy meals, and result in "poor" dietary decisions. I am using quotation marks here because our bodies assume that we need more readily available energy during times of stress, which junk food has plenty of. On top of all this, stress is harmful for the digestive system. It raises triglycerides and impairs the motility of the stomach and intestines. Impaired activation of the vagus nerve, which also influences insulin response, is behind this. The vagus nerve is a cranial nerve that controls muscle contractions and enzyme production in the digestive system.

Cultures across the world have linked emotional health to the physical body for centuries. Even though they are thousands of kilometres apart, both Chinese medicine (TCM) and people in the Meru region of Kenya have traditionally described anger as a liver problem. My friend Kageni Njeru, Soul Coach and "energy engineer", explains that if someone was angry all the time, they would say "That person has a rotten liver". If you met a cruel bully, you would say "That person has a rotten heart", or you would describe someone as having a bad tongue if they were the jealous, gossiping type. In a small village, this could earn you a bad reputation quickly.

Besides general stress, shame can cause inflammation too. In a 2004 study of 49 people, some were asked to write about traumatic experiences where they blamed themselves, while others wrote about neutral experiences. Both inflammatory markers and emotional responses were measured before and after each of the three writing sessions. Those in the self-blame group showed higher levels of guilt and shame, as well as higher levels of inflammation. Greater levels of shame were linked with greater increases in inflammation, but guilt and general negative emotions seemed to be unrelated. This is why I strongly advise against shaming anyone with an inflammatory or neurological disorder – they are adults who need healing, not children or a source of comedy because of their potentially embarrassing health issues.

Sadly, menstruation is a source of shame and other negative emotions for many women and girls. In *From Menstrual Shame to Bleeding as a Spiritual Practice*, a chapter of *The Psychology of Shame: New Research*, author Sharon Moloney describes interviewing Australian women with varying attitudes towards menstruation. One woman went from joining in with the culture of shame so prevalent at her high school, to honouring the menstrual cycle as sacred in her thirties. Others stated:

Alexandra Preston

"I got my periods when I was 14 and I was just so embarrassed!"

"I was embarrassed going to the toilets at school and having to change pads and realising that if I came out, the girls outside would know what I'd been doing."

"When I was at high school, we had an incinerator in the toilet, so there was the shame of coming out after the puff of smoke went up. The boys would check who came out and then you'd get the name-calling, sometimes from other girls as well."

"One time we were at the beach and she (Mum) was so ashamed that I was bleeding. I was eleven, having my second period, and she rushed me to the toilet and cursed me the whole way."

"My mother never spoke to me about it; she was too embarrassed. She'd grown up as a strict Baptist and had very repressed ideas around sex."

Besides shame, negative attitudes towards menstruation in general can cause, and be a result of, period pain and PMS. A study on mindfulness found that women who described their periods as "debilitating" or "bothersome" reported more premenstrual pain. However, women with higher mindfulness scores in non-judging, non-reacting, observing and describing had less severe symptoms on average.

Menstrual shame has no place in a woman's life; we can see this by how many have been hurt by such attitudes. Not

Infla-Menses

only is it inflammatory, but some indigenous American cultures see shame as a block to spiritual growth. The best remedy is practicing poise, self-pride, personal power and self-acceptance.

Even if motherhood isn't something you want in life, remember that menstrual blood contains stem cells too! I first learnt that by accident when I was 17. From then onwards, I stopped feeling like my menstrual cycle was an unwanted inconvenience, as healing people has always been far more meaningful to me than adding another baby to the world. While menstrual stem cells are unfortunately under-researched compared to other types, *Parent's Guide to Cord Blood* lists over 80 conditions that stem cells in general are approved for (as at least part of mainstream treatment) at the time of writing this book. Also as of mid-2019, there are Phase 3 clinical trials testing stem cells for osteoarthritis, Motor Neuron Disease and other issues. These are using bone marrow stem cells, while one advantage of menstrual stem cells is that no needles are required to extract them, just a cup. Even if they turn out to be less effective than other stem cell types, the presence of stem cells in menstrual blood can still be symbolic of restoration and renewal.

What Can We Do About It?

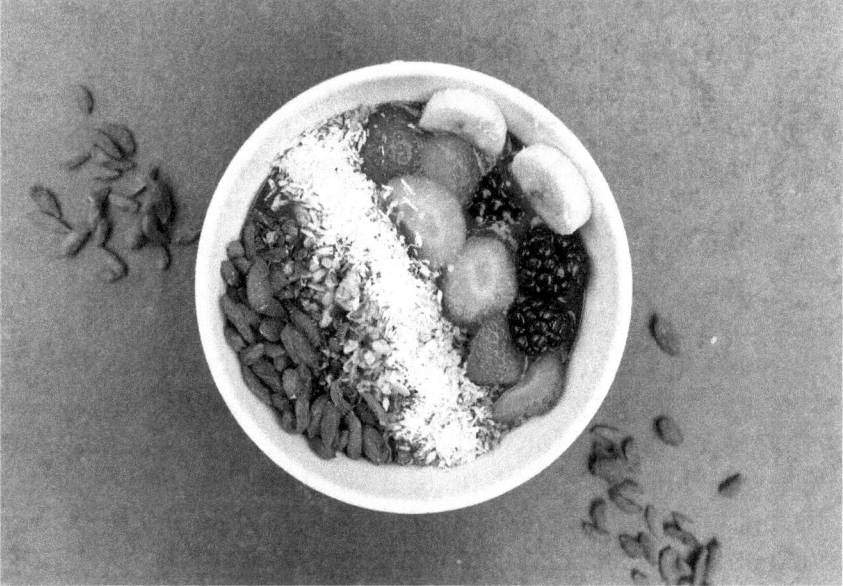

In a nutshell, an anti-inflammatory diet is one of your best defences against period pain and PMS when they are triggered by inflammation. This emphasises whole, organic (if possible) foods, i.e. vegetables, fruits, wholegrains, beans, legumes, nuts, seeds and oily fish. Red meat, dairy, processed foods, fried foods, refined carbohydrates, sugar and alcohol are meant to be reduced or eliminated. It is very similar to a diet you'd go on if you were focusing on reducing glycation, or the opposite of a modern Western diet. As for supplementation, however, please only take this as a guide in case of any contraindications. Particularly if you have a chronic illness and are on medication (hormonal contraception counts as medication too), it is best to see a qualified professional one-on-one before taking supplements or significantly changing your diet.

If you have an inflammatory condition such as endometriosis, you may first want to test your levels of inflammatory markers to see where you're at now and how well you are improving with holistic treatment. The best common tests, according to Dr Dale Bredesen, are hs-CRP, TNF-a and IL-6. CRP is made by the liver in response to inflammation. It is best to test high-sensitivity CRP (hs-CRP) because normal CRP isn't always accurate enough. Interleukin-6 (IL-6) and tumour necrosis factor-alpha (TNF-a) are inflammatory immune chemicals. If your immune system was a police force, they or the cells that produce them would be like dispatchers. If you test your omega-6 to -3 ratio, it should be less than 3, but more than 0.5 (too much omega-3 fats can cause haemorrhage; avoid this).

The Importance of a Holistic Approach

Why should we see a professional who can help us take a holistic approach to healing, instead of trying out different diets to see what works or whatever supplement is currently getting the most attention? Well, there is no one "magic pill" to give us all a healthy menstrual cycle without much effort. There are thousands of physiological processes going on in the body every day, and every month, all interrelated in a complex web that can terrify most new naturopathy or Ayurveda students. This is why the "one manmade chemical to hammer one pathway" approach of pharmaceutical medicine often causes many negative side effects in exchange for a few benefits (if it works at all!). It is also why the seemingly milder effects of herbs or dietary supplements are safer and more effective when used correctly. Physiological pathways are more likely to be modulated than blocked or ramped up, so the downstream effects are less likely to cause harm.

Even just one whole herb or nutrient can benefit multiple processes, with the many phytochemicals in each herb strengthening, modulating, changing or adding to the effects of each other. However, systems of natural medicine have used holistic protocols for thousands of years, in order to target as many causes and effects of a problem as possible. One plant may be easier to remember – especially before literacy – but holistic protocols have always been worth it, because they work!

Let's look at my profession, naturopathy, as an example. When treating a client, we use diet advice; lifestyle changes; nutritional supplements; herbal medicine; homeopathy; and sometimes, depending on our training, other natural therapies such as massage, hydrotherapy or energy healing. My extra therapies are flower essence therapy, Emotional Freedom Technique (EFT) and energy healing using the Diamond frequency.

On the 20th of February, 2019, a review of 33 studies found that naturopathy as a whole system is effective for a range of chronic conditions, such as cardiovascular disease, depression, anxiety, diabetes, musculoskeletal pain and polycystic ovarian syndrome (PCOS). In the case of PCOS, one of the Australian studies compared personalised lifestyle plans, with life coaching, both alone and in combination with

Infla-Menses

herbal medicine prescriptions. After three months, women in the combined treatment group recorded a 32.9% reduction in oligomenorrhoea compared to the lifestyle-only group. On average, menstrual cycle length was a staggering 43 days shorter in the women given herbal medicine. They also enjoyed improvements in BMI, blood pressure, depression, anxiety, quality of life, luteinising hormone and fertility.

Additionally, a cohort study of 60 from the USA looked at the benefits of naturopathy for depression and anxiety, two common manifestations of PMS, or tag-along pests that accompany other chronic health issues. The most common therapies used were nutritional supplements, herbal medicine, homeopathy and acupuncture. After at least two visits, depression and anxiety symptoms were reduced by an average of 48% and 42%, respectively, which is similar to my own results in practice. Even though these studies did not use the same intervention for everyone like clinical trials for pharmaceutical drugs, they examined how naturopathy is used in the real world.

Dietary Interventions

A Plant-Based Diet

While too much meat can contribute to inflammation, a mostly or totally vegetarian diet can be very effective in relieving it. In a study involving 31 overweight and obese volunteers, all were instructed to follow a strict vegetarian diet for four weeks, which was meant to be vegan and mostly raw. After the month, not only did their mean BMI fall from 37 to 35 (a BMI of over 30 is classified as obese), but their levels of key inflammatory markers dropped considerably. I still recommend cooked foods such as bean and lentil dishes, as they often have more protein and less antinutrients. In the Blue Zones – regions with the highest lifespans and healthspans – Dan Buettner noted that meat is typically consumed up to five times per month. As I wrote above, age-related diseases are inflammatory too; you just notice menstrual problems much earlier.

General Health

It seems like everyone I know is turning vegetarian or vegan. As someone with an interest in natural, holistic life extension, I had to ask the question: do vegetarian and vegan diets help people live longer? If so, that means they benefit our overall health, and do not simply substitute one awful set of illnesses and degeneration for another. It turns out that they are beneficial for longevity, as long as you do it right.

In the USA, Michael J. Orlich and colleagues at Loma Linda University, California, analysed the mortality rates of 73,308 people from the US and Canada in the Adventist Health Study-2 (AHS-2), who were tracked for six years. They were divided into five groups: meat eaters, semi-vegetarians, pescatarians, vegetarians and vegans. When all types of vegetarians were grouped together, their average adjusted risk of dying during the study period was 12% lower than that of meat eaters. Vegan men had a 28% lower risk of dying over the almost six-year period. While some will tell you that vegetarians and vegans only seem healthier because they are less likely to smoke and drink, and are more health-conscious, active and educated, most people in the AHS-2 study fit this description regardless of their diet.

Infla-Menses

Over in the UK, the EPIC Oxford cohort, involving over sixty thousand people, found no significant longevity benefits. Those in the EPIC cohort consumed less fibre and vitamin C than the AHS-2 participants, as they were more likely to be what was described as the "pudding and cake" type of vegetarian (i.e. where frozen pizza is in, quinoa and lentils are out). The reduced risk of dying from cancer only appeared after nearly 15 years of a vegetarian diet. Not all vegetarian diets are created equal, but lower rates of disease and mortality linked to being vegetarian are "one of the most consistent findings of nutritional epidemiology", according to Dr David Jacobs, PhD and Mayo professor of epidemiology. Yet more evidence even came out while I was writing this book! A study of over twelve thousand people, followed for years, found that those in the top fifth for plant food consumption had a 32% lower cardiovascular disease death rate and a 25% lower risk of dying from any cause in a given time.

A plant-based diet looks like the best way to optimise your intestinal microbiome. When omnivorous volunteers were put on a lacto-ovo vegetarian diet for three months, it began to change the gut bacteria composition and immune balance. While there wasn't enough time to create major changes to species diversity, species with known beneficial effects, such as butyrate producers and some linked with IgA antibodies, were increased. There were also fewer T-cell types, less IgE expression, and few inflammation-related genes in the gut flora among the long-term vegetarians. IgA antibodies are made to protect the tissues, while IgE antibodies are used in the inflammatory response. Therefore, increased IgA may mean a less leaky gut.

As for specific species, high numbers of one known as *Firmicutes prausnitzii* have been associated with lower inflammation. This species, found in higher populations among vegans, is one of the anti-inflammatory short-chain fatty acid (SCFA) producers. Optimal levels of SCFAs can also improve cardiovascular health and reduce your risk of diabetes later on.

As we now know, lipopolysaccharides are involved in endometriosis development. The above study found that only long-term vegetarians had significantly lower expression of LPS-related genes in their intestinal microbiome. That means you shouldn't give up if you have endometriosis and are only slowly improving on a vegetarian diet! Always ensure that you are getting enough nutrients, but don't let smug steak-lovers get you down because you or they didn't expect healing to take this long.

Do you have PCOS and are struggling to lose weight? A small study of six obese, diabetic volunteers found that going vegan for one month significantly reduced body weight, excess blood glucose and levels of glycation (as I wrote above, plant-based meals are lower in AGEs). Their vegan diet also cut down populations of a bacteria "family", called *Enterobacteriaceae* in the scientific world, which triggers low-grade inflammation. This low-grade inflammation is particularly problematic, as we usually aren't aware that we have it until chronic health issues appear. The higher fibre content of vegan diets is thought to be the largest contributor to these anti-inflammatory changes in gut bacteria, so if you can't or don't want to be vegan, increasing the proportions of vegetables, wholegrains and legumes can still help.

Another involved 74 people with type II diabetes, who were randomly assigned to either a conventional anti-diabetic diet or a vegetarian one, high in vegetables, fruit, nuts, grains, legumes and seeds. The only animal food allowed was one portion of low-fat yoghurt a day, making it almost vegan. Although both diets had the same caloric restriction, the vegetarian diet was twice as effective in reducing body weight, resulting in an average of 6.2kg of weight lost compared to 3.2kg.

It wasn't simply weight loss either. Using magnetic resonance imaging (MRI), the doctors performing this study then looked at how fat tissue was stored in the patients' thighs. Fat tissue in our limbs can be stored under the skin (subcutaneous), on the surface of muscles (subfascial) and inside the muscles (intramuscular). Both diets resulted in a similar reduction in subcutaneous fat. However, only the vegetarian diet reduced subfascial fat, and was far more effective in reducing the amount of intramuscular fat. Why is this important? Subfascial fat is associated with insulin resistance in type II diabetes, so reducing it could benefit sugar metabolism in ways that just any old weight loss cannot. Reducing intramuscular fat could also help to improve muscle strength and mobility, which is particularly important in older people.

Other research has shown that being vegan is linked to lower risks of some autoimmune conditions, which are characterised by inflammation so dysregulated that the immune system attacks parts of the human body. For example, a study on Seventh-Day Adventists found that only a vegan diet was associated with the prevention of hypothyroidism, not vegetarian diets.

Clinical trials also demonstrate improvement in rheumatoid arthritis, where the immune system attacks the joints. One, involving 53 patients participating in a year-long shift from a conventional diet to a vegan and later a lacto-vegetarian diet, found significant changes in gut bacteria too. Those with the greatest improvements in their disease had a greater shift towards an anti-inflammatory bacteria profile. A second trial tested a raw vegan diet, which is quite extreme as food cannot be heated past 42 degrees. Only the vegan group enjoyed a reduced disease activity in some volunteers.

Menstrual Health

When it comes to menstrual problems specifically, while red meat has been linked to double the risk of an endometriosis diagnosis, higher green vegetable consumption is related to a 70% lower chance of diagnosis! Eating more fruit is associated with a 40% smaller risk. It's also important to consume unprocessed foods. Switching saturated and monounsaturated fats for trans-fat was, in the same study, linked to a 20% higher risk of the disease, and trading omega-3s for trans-fat doubled their danger. Changing from trans fats to these resulted in the opposite effect, i.e. switching to omega-3 fats halved their risk. Avocadoes and olive oil are two examples of monounsaturated fat sources. I recommend keeping olive oil to salads and dips, as unsaturated fats may become unstable when heated in a manner such as frying (I use coconut oil as it is stable).

Infla-Menses

A vegetarian diet may help to reduce dysmenorrhoea too. In a crossover study, 33 women followed a low-fat vegetarian diet for two menstrual cycles, and then took a placebo supplement for another two cycles while following their usual diet. The average number of days that they had cramping fell from 3.9 to 2.7 while on the vegetarian diet, but it went back to normal once they went on the placebo pill. Average pain intensity and certain PMS symptoms, including water retention and concentration, also fell significantly.

These effects were mainly attributed to higher levels of sex hormone binding globulin (SHBG), which holds onto sex hormones such as oestrogen so they don't do more than necessary. However, inflammation is linked with lower SHBG in both menstruating and post-menopausal women; therefore going vegetarian would benefit both inflammation and hormone balance. It may be helpful too if you have a young daughter and are worried about early puberty! More plant-based diets have been linked to later age at menarche, most likely because of less free sex hormones.

I am not saying that you as an individual must go vegan or vegetarian full-time in order to reduce inflammation, but you are likely to benefit from reducing your intake of red meat and poultry, such as by being vegetarian for a couple of days per week. However, an increasing number of people are going vegetarian, vegan, pescatarian (fish and shellfish are permitted, but no red meat or poultry) or flexitarian (part-time vegetarian), especially younger women, so I needed to discuss:

Preventing Deficiencies in a Plant-Based Diet

In what has traditionally been a meat-and-three-veg society, common concerns when going vegetarian are how to get enough of nutrients such as protein, iron and zinc. These are an issue when cutting down on red meat, but strict vegetarians can also become deficient in omega-3 fats, vitamin B12, vitamin K2 and vitamin A without the correct information. Remember that inflammation causes iron deficiency, so if red meat makes you inflamed, well-meaning advice from meat-loving relatives may not work.

Protein

"But where will you get your protein?" is the most common question that full-time meat eaters ask vegetarians and vegans. This, however, may be the easiest problem to solve. A French study on over ninety-three thousand people found that vegetarians were more likely than vegans or meat eaters to fall within the recommended protein intake, at 73.8%. Over one quarter of meat eaters and one in ten vegetarians in fact ate too much protein. Excessive protein intake is not recommended unless you are trying to build a considerable amount of muscle, or (in some cases) you are recovering from injury or surgery. Most vegetarians and vegans in the study were therefore able to successfully substitute meat for plant protein sources such as beans and legumes.

Iron

Younger women are at greater risk of iron-deficiency anaemia because of menstruation, but there are ways around it! While iron from meat and other animal products has a 15-35% absorption rate, it drops to 2-20% for plant sources due to the presence of antinutrients, which reduce absorption of minerals such as iron, calcium and zinc. Vitamin C, however, cancels out their effects and helps to enhance absorption, so it's important to eat fresh fruits and vegetables – not just microwaveable vegetarian frozen dinners. Sprouting or soaking grains, legumes and nuts helps to break down and remove antinutrients too. As for green leafy vegetables, they should be cooked, such as by steaming or blanching. Finally, avoiding tea or coffee close to meals is advisable as some of their phytochemicals impair iron absorption.

How much iron do we need? Women with a menstrual cycle should aim for around 18mg of iron per day, as opposed to 8mg for people who don't have one. Vegetarian protein sources are some of the best ways to get iron too: lentils contain an average of 4.1-4.9mg per ¾ cup, while black, pinto, kidney and white beans have anywhere from 2.6 to 4.9 mg per ¾ cup (all cooked). Tempeh has around 3.2mg of iron per 150 gram serving. As for vegetables, cooked spinach and tomato puree contain 2-3.4mg and 2.4mg per half cup respectively, while asparagus has 2.1mg per six spears. Per ounce (28 grams), SELF's *Nutrition Data* lists the iron content of pepitas at 4.2mg.

Zinc
Another mineral to watch out for if you're going vegetarian or reducing meat is zinc. Women need around 8mg of zinc per day, less than men. One quarter-cup of pumpkin seeds gives 2.3mg of zinc; the same amount of cashews and sunflower seeds yields 1.9mg and 1.7mg respectively. Half a cup of tofu has around 2mg, and cooked lentils and chickpeas each have 1.3mg per half cup.

Nutritional yeast, which you can add to vegan cheese, contains 2mg per tablespoon. Tahini has roughly 1.5mg per tablespoon.

Calcium
If you are avoiding all dairy foods, the best sources of calcium are, according to the Seattle Children's Hospital, sardines (unless you are totally vegan), firm tofu with the nigari, and rhubarb listed as "cooked with sugar". These all contain over 200mg per serving. Homemade baked beans, blackstrap molasses, cooked spinach, amaranth, tahini, turnip greens, collard greens and quinoa have at least 100mg per serve. Kale, almond butter, almonds, chickpeas, figs and bok choy contain over 75mg per serving. Plant sources should be cooked in order to remove the antinutrients that prevent calcium absorption.

If you would miss milk, and not just the calcium in it, there is a wide range of commercially available plant milks, such as almond, hemp and coconut milk. *Mind Over Munch* also has a helpful video tutorial on how to make your own plant-based milks, including strawberry coconut milk, cinnamon rice milk and blueberry hemp milk. I prefer to buy organic plant milks that have been enriched with plant-derived calcium, so I am not missing out on what is most important.

How Teff Can Help
One very interesting gluten-free grain, teff, is particularly rich in protein, iron, zinc and calcium compared to other grains. This plant comes from Ethiopia and surrounding countries in the Horn of Africa, and is thought to get its name from the Amharic word *teffa*, meaning "lost", as its

seeds are so small. Traditionally, it is ground into flour which is then fermented overnight in water and fried to make the flatbread known as *injera*. Some health food stores sell teff flour, with other ideas on their packaging such as (quite dense) pancakes.

The protein content of teff is roughly 11%, comparable to wheat and barley and higher than rice or maize. However, the predominant types of protein in teff are also easier to digest. Compared to these grains, teff is the richest source of the amino acids alanine and histidine, the building blocks of carnosine. As I wrote in *High-AGE Foods*, carnosine plays an important role in preventing glycation but is only present in red meat; vegetarians must make their own. It is very high in iron, with an estimated 15.7mg per 100g of grains, and has 4.8mg per 100g of zinc. This almost meets the iron requirements of an average woman with a menstrual cycle, and over half of a woman's zinc requirements. Additionally, teff contains 165mg of calcium and 180mg of magnesium per 100g, making it a healthy vegan source of calcium and a much-needed source of magnesium for everyone, as deficiency is common.

Vitamin A

Another common deficiency among vegetarians and vegans is that of vitamin A, as pre-formed vitamin A is only found in animal products. Under 10% of the over 600 carotenoids can be converted to vitamin A, including beta-carotene, lutein, lycopene, canthaxanthin and zeaxanthin. Beta-carotene has the highest rate of conversion, at roughly 50%. Red, orange and yellow vegetables and fruits contain high levels of carotenoids, such as carrots, squash, pumpkin, rockmelon, tomatoes and watermelon (lycopene is the red pigment in these two). Green vegetables have some carotenoids, but you can't see them because of the chlorophyll.

Spirulina, however, has demonstrated a high conversion rate of its beta-carotene content. Studies in areas where vitamin A deficiency is particularly prevalent have found that spirulina is just as effective as pure vitamin A in raising its levels back to the healthy range. One of these involved women living by Lake Chad, an overall low-income region where nutritional deficiencies are common. Spirulina grows naturally in some areas of the lake, and is prepared by people of the Kanembou ethnicity into a powder called *dihé*. In other words, this is a traditional food – not a trendy hipster ingredient for privileged models or personal trainers, not a standardised supplement specifically formulated to produce a specific result for an experiment out to prove that we don't need meat or GMOs.

When women who ate *dihé* at least three times per week (mostly Kanembou women) were compared to those who didn't eat it (mostly Arab women), their blood levels of vitamin A were higher. Due to living in the same area and having a relatively small range of food choices, their diets were not significantly different. Their high consumption of peanut oil also tells us to not be fat-phobic, as the fats in olives and nuts aid conversion of beta-carotene to vitamin A.

Vitamin K

Vitamin K is an issue too, but it's not as bad as some would make it out to be. There are two major forms in food: vitamin K1 in plants, and K2 in animal products and natto, a strong-smelling, Japanese fermented soy food. It could be worth developing an acquired taste, as natto contains over 100 times more K2 than the cheeses it is found in, and can improve bone health in older women. We need K2 to help chaperone calcium to the bones and away from the blood vessels, among other purposes.

But if you can't stand or buy natto and are vegan, is there a way to get the vitamin without taking supplements? A study involving breastfeeding mothers divided them into four groups of different vitamin K1 doses, and measured their milk levels of K2 over two and a half weeks. It didn't have much of an effect on day 4, but on day 16 they were producing dramatically higher levels of K2 from the supplemental plant form. Leafy green vegetables and some fruits contain vitamin K1, such as kale, Brussels sprouts, spinach, broccoli, mustard greens and asparagus.

Vitamin B12
If you are vegetarian, you can still get small amounts of vitamin B12 from eggs, dairy and dirty vegetables (not exactly recommended). If you decide to eat fish at least occasionally, sardines are particularly high in the vitamin, with *Nutrition Data* reporting B12 content at 8.2 micrograms per 92g can. This is over the recommended intake of 2.4 micrograms. However, research suggests that tempeh contains a significant amount of vitamin B12, at 0.7-0.8 micrograms/100g, and so do some species of seaweed (dried green laver, or *Enteromorpha spp.*, and nori/purple laver, *Porphyra spp.*). Fermenting vegetables with certain species of lactic acid-producing or propionic bacteria can boost levels of the vitamin too. A few species of edible mushrooms have also registered significant levels of B12, in particular shiitake (*Lentinula edodes*), black trumpet (*Craterellus*

cornucopioides) and golden chanterelle (*Cantharellus cibarius*). The study on shiitake mushrooms revealed that this came from the bed logs they were grown on. Therefore, in a world where vegetarian and vegan diets are common, we would ideally ensure that our shiitake mushrooms are grown on logs with B12-producing bacteria, and that vegetables are fermented with them too.

Carnosine

Besides vitamin B12, the only nutrient we cannot get from a vegetarian diet is carnosine. Carnosine plays a key role in reducing the harmful glycation reactions which are known to be responsible for so much of aging. But how do the animals that give us carnosine through food obtain it themselves? Carnosine is made of the amino acids beta-alanine and L-histidine, and research on older adults (55-92) does show that beta-alanine supplementation improves physical working capacity. Additionally, sprint training increases the level of carnosine in muscle. Just like herbivorous animals, we make carnosine ourselves.

The Low-FODMAP Diet

Sometimes, including in many cases of IBS, we have too many intestinal bacteria and need to temporarily reduce carbohydrate intake. A key similarity between endometriosis and IBS is visceral hypersensitivity, where the body is over-sensitive to pain and inflammation. In a New Zealand study, 36% of the 160 women with IBS also had endometriosis. On a low FODMAP diet, 72% with endometriosis reported a more than 50% improvement in bowel symptoms after a month, compared to 49% without the disease.

Infla-Menses

FODMAPs are short-chain carbohydrates (including some sugars) that are not absorbed well, and usually feed intestinal bacteria. They are Fermentable; Oligosaccharides, short-chain carbs seen in wheat, rye, onions, garlic and legumes; Disaccharides, in other words lactose from dairy; Monosaccharides, in this case fructose from honey and fruit; and Polyols, which are used as artificial sweeteners but found in some fruit and vegetables.

A low FODMAP diet is not meant to be followed forever, only for about two or three months. This is enough time to reduce the overpopulated gut microbiome, but not so much that it becomes underpopulated and you lose too many beneficial species. It is also difficult to follow if you are vegetarian or vegan. High FODMAP foods include legumes, mushrooms and stone fruits; while low FODMAP, permissible foods include seafood, green vegetables and citrus fruits. You can find the most comprehensive database of forbidden and permissible foods with the Monash University FODMAP Diet App.

You can start reintroducing FODMAPS after around six weeks, one food at a time every three days while carefully watching for any reactions. Most people will be able to eat some high-FODMAP foods, and will have to avoid others. One of my patients had to spend a few months on a low FODMAP diet, and eventually was able to eat moderate amounts of previously harmful foods like chickpeas. As a vegan, I had to assist them in finding the right foods so they wouldn't suffer from deficiencies during this time.

The Ketogenic Diet

The ketogenic diet defies the very mid-20th century idea that fat makes you, well, fat, and always causes cardiovascular disease. The truth is, as Dr Uffe Ravnskov, MD and PhD, stated in 2008: "The diet heart hypothesis is sustained by social, political and financial institutions which have little to do with science and established success in public health". Many people benefit from high-fat diets, and in some cases the ketogenic diet is their best option. To be effective, it requires a ratio of fats to protein and carbohydrates of 4:1, or at least 3:1. The "classic" keto diet aims for 90% fat, 6% protein and 4% carbs; modified keto aims for 82% fat, 12% protein and 6% carbs; and the MCT keto diet allows for 73% fat, 10% protein and 17% carbs, provided that highly-ketogenic medium-chain triglycerides are consumed.

The ketogenic diet works by pushing the body to use the breakdown products of fats, known as ketones, for energy instead of sugar. It has been used since 1923 in epilepsy, and may aid other neurological problems such as brain injury and autism as well as some mitochondrial disorders. In my experience, I have helped to shift menopausal weight gain with the ketogenic diet. If you are interested in going keto, I recommend that you do it in cycles (one small study on autism used it four weeks on, two weeks off) and consult a qualified health professional face-to-face, as there are some contraindications and risks that must be managed. Some people have modified the ketogenic diet to be vegan or vegetarian, which would help to shift the fat composition to an anti-inflammatory one. I advise against the steak, bacon and eggs interpretation; it is not friendly to the heart, immune system or wallet.

If you suffer from menstrual problems, the ketogenic diet may be an effective way to reduce inflammation, particularly if you also have a neurological or metabolic condition and only if it is safe for you. Using ketones for energy produces less oxidative free radicals, making it easier for the antioxidants in your body to protect you against damage. Less oxidative damage can mean less inflammation. Clinical studies have shown that a ketogenic diet can reduce inflammation, relieving inflamed livers in people with non-alcoholic fatty liver disease.

Additionally, a study on 83 obese people found that strictly following the diet for 24 weeks led to an average weight loss of 14.36 kilograms, far better than the above study. In another, 64 obese people followed a ketogenic diet for 56 weeks (around one year and one month). Thirty-one of them had type II diabetes. After these 56 weeks, those with diabetes lost around 24 kilograms, and those with normal blood sugar levels lost about 30 kilograms on average. In other happy news for the diabetic volunteers, their blood sugar levels dropped into the normal range! And in both of these studies, the weight loss was sustained; they did not gain it back.

Does this mean the ketogenic diet can help with PCOS? In a pilot study of 11 women (only five completed it), they were all instructed to follow a keto diet with 20 grams or less of carbohydrates per day for 24 weeks. Those who finished the diet plan enjoyed a 12% decrease in body weight, a 22% drop in free testosterone, a 36% drop in LH/FSH ratio and a

54% fall in fasting insulin. Two even became pregnant despite suffering infertility in the past. There were also some improvements in the menstrual cycle, body hair and blood sugar control.

The Paleo Diet

In Australia, the Paleo diet is associated with social media stars and celebrity chefs, then promptly belittled for being a trendy "fad". The Paleo diet aims to copy the eating patterns of pre-agricultural societies. It includes vegetables, fruit, eggs and meat, usually nuts and seeds, and sometimes certain grains and legumes, typically soaked or sprouted. Dairy, processed foods and most grains are forbidden. Like the ketogenic diet, some people follow a vegetarian, vegan or pescatarian version, and you can do it in a cyclic pattern.

Despite being mocked in the media, there is research to back it up, including studies on its anti-inflammatory benefits. Seventy post-menopausal women, with an average age of 60, followed either a Paleo diet or "prudent" control diet for two years to see if it was superior to generic advice. Abdominal fat decreased significantly more in the Paleo group over the first six months, and this was maintained at 24 months. Inflammatory gene expression was positively affected, showing diet-by-time interactions and persistent benefits.

In my own practice, I have seen older women more or less requiring a Paleo or low-carb diet, at least temporarily, if they want to lose inflammatory post-menopausal weight. This study also shows that there's no shame in wanting to lose menopausal weight just to look good – there are side benefits! Who cares what our Stone Age ancestors really ate, as long as it works! A rose is a rose by any other name. As aging is linked to runaway inflammation, if it benefits 60 year old women, it's likely to benefit you in your 20s or 30s.

The Paleo diet is certainly not your mother's or grandmother's diet. There is evidence that acne is so often caused by a high glycaemic load-diet, where dairy, grains (at least the refined ones) and refined sugars drive up your blood sugar. Milk can make the effects of refined grains even worse than what they would be left alone. The resulting increase in insulin, insulin-like growth factor 1 (IGF-1) and insulin resistance both harm your internal health and trigger pathways that cause acne. In a nutshell, they make certain glands in your skin too friendly to *Propionibacterium acnes*, the main microbial driver of acne.

On the other hand, low glycaemic eating patterns such as the Paleo diet can significantly reduce the number of inflammatory and non-inflammatory acne spots. The effects on insulin sensitivity also mean that going Paleo may help if you have PCOS. I noticed the benefits of a low-glycaemic load diet myself on a client of mine with acne. Over four thousand dollars' worth of cosmetic treatments barely dented her skin problems, but reducing her glycaemic load (especially in the morning) meant next to no new spots!

If you are vegetarian or vegan, making low-carb diets more difficult, some practitioners recommend timing carbohydrate restriction to the phases of the menstrual cycle. During the luteal phase, around day 15-28 of the menstrual cycle (or after ovulation, but before menstruation), high progesterone and lower oestrogen reduces insulin sensitivity.

Therefore, this is the best time to restrict carbs if you only want to go keto or Paleo sometimes.

Intermittent Fasting

Intermittent fasting is when you limit your food intake to a certain number of hours every day. This is typically within 8-12 hours, without restricting the number of kilojoules to a dangerous level. Some people eat normally most days, but choose certain days to fast. My Muslim friends do this in a way during Ramadan, and one gym buddy of mine actually says she feels great and still goes to all her usual morning classes! With intermittent fasting, you do it most days of the year instead of one month, and the hours are more sustainable to support this.

What can it do for inflammatory health problems? Some of intermittent fasting's effects come from its ability to increase the intestinal microbiome diversity. *Lactobacillaceae*, *Bacteroidaceae* and *Prevotellaceae* populations all rose in mice. It also shifted the balance of the immune system to a more inflammation-regulating state, as opposed to a pro-inflammatory one. When the same researchers tested an intermittent fasting protocol in humans with MS, their levels of inflammation fell while microbial diversity rose. The types of bacteria encouraged by this protocol, where they fasted every second day, produce anti-inflammatory short-chained fats and are known to be reduced in patients with MS. The short study period – just two weeks – wasn't long enough to see any differences in disability scores.

Intermittent fasting doesn't just improve the intestinal microbiome. Other research has found that it can reduce glycation, with reductions of 1.0 or more units being reported. One comparing two methods demonstrated that fasting (consuming only 25% of usual energy intake) for five days, once every five weeks, was more effective than fasting one day per week. It also improves mitochondrial health – they produce energy for our cells – by boosting production of new mitochondria and recycling those too damaged to continue on. The recycling of damaged cellular parts is called autophagy. When this is impaired, cells become dysfunctional and create more damage and inflammation. Fasting is like calling in housekeeping.

Impaired autophagy may contribute to endometriosis. A lab study of tissue samples from patients found that a drug used to enhance the process actually reduced the invasive qualities of endometriotic cells. Another on 36 women with PCOS looked at their expression of genes related to autophagy. The women with PCOS had a lower expression of autophagy-related genes in their uterine lining compared to healthy women. However, when some took metformin (pharmaceutical medicine's way of fixing the problem), their function was somewhat restored. This drug does have side effects, while intermittent fasting and other natural interventions have side-benefits. Unless you cannot fast and must use something else, you would also strengthen your *mental muscles* in terms of self-control and delayed gratification.

Going Organic

In the previous section of this book, I described some nasty effects of the thousands of toxins currently used in today's world. One way to reduce your exposure and support health-promoting practices is to go organic where possible. Organic food contains far lower levels of toxins such as pesticides, and is more likely to have no residues. However, it isn't completely free of them (yet) because of pesticide drift and remaining contamination from when the land was used for conventional farming.

Organic food can have higher levels of some nutrients too. Multiple studies have shown that organic produce is richer in vitamin C, phosphorous, iron, magnesium and phytochemicals with antioxidant effects. For example, organic grapes had higher levels of resveratrol and total polyphenols (an antioxidant class of phytochemicals). Organic potatoes had more vitamin C and chlorogenic acid, which is also responsible for much of coffee's antioxidant effect. Organically grown foods may increase in some areas of nutritional value as the land "matures", which takes years. As for all this translating to health benefits, one study involving toddlers has even shown that those eating organic dairy products have a 36% lower risk of eczema.

If you are transitioning to an organic diet, it is best to search online for the best deals on quality and price. Global chains like Aldi stock growing ranges of organic foods, and there may be smaller delivery services in your local area, such as Ripe n Raw Organics in Southeast Queensland. Farmers markets can be a great way to meet producers you can trust.

If you can, growing some of your own food is a rewarding way to help yourself go organic. You don't need a large amount of land, except if you aim to grow most of your food or want an impressive food forest. These are

Infla-Menses

increasingly popular from American survivalists to villages working with Ecosia in Senegal. Instead, you can grow a container garden; even if you live in an apartment, not everything is off-limits. Water and light exposure are necessary considerations, and so is root depth. A useful guide I found by Preparedness Mama outlines what you can grow in a four, six, eight or 12 inch pot (in Australia, this is 10, 15, 20 and 30 centimetres).

Root Depth	Suitable Foods
Four inches/ 10cm	Asian greens, garlic, marjoram, mint, mustard, radishes, salad greens, thyme.
Six inches/ 15cm	All of the above, basil, bush beans, chervil, chives, coriander, dill, lettuce, nasturtium, onion, oregano, peas, pole beans, round carrots, shallots, runner beans, spinach, strawberries, zucchini.
Eight inches/ 20cm	All of the above, cabbage, chard, capsicum (bell pepper), chillies, cucumber, eggplant, fava bean, fennel, kale, leek, some melons, parsley, parsnips, pumpkin, rosemary, sage, squash, tarragon, tomato, turnip.
12 inches/ 30cm	All of the above, bay, beetroot, blueberry, carrots, corn, currants, fruit trees (at least dwarf varieties), gooseberries, kiwifruit, potatoes, raspberries, rhubarb.

Remember that pots and containers need more frequent watering, especially non-glazed ceramics. Darker colours are better for shadier areas too. This is by no means a gardening book, just an introduction to what you can do with limited space. Don't hesitate to look for comprehensive information on vertical and container gardening.

If you have the space for it, a forest garden replicates the ways that plants thrive in nature without toxic products such as pesticides. Different species provide each other with nutrients, moisture and all-round protection while aiding soil health and biodiversity. They are also far more productive than monocultures.

Eat Your Fruit and Vegetables

It's no surprise that eating a broad range of fruits and vegetables helps to reduce inflammation and balance your menstrual cycle. In a very large women's health study, for example, eating citrus fruits at least once per week was linked to a 22% lower risk of endometriosis. Having avocadoes one to three times weekly decreased their risk by 37%. Another on university students in the UAE found a 66% lower chance of PMS symptoms interfering with daily life if the women regularly ate fruit. Specific fruits and vegetables that can be of benefit in menstrual problems are pineapple, pomegranates, cruciferous vegetables, moringa and red grapes (resveratrol).

Bromelain (Pineapple)

It turns out that one super phytochemical unfortunately gets thrown away all the time. Bromelain is a mix of protein-digesting enzymes found in certain fruits, including pineapple cores. At a therapeutic dose, it has been shown to help relieve inflammatory diseases such as arthritis and IBD. Bromelain achieves this by several pathways that may involve arachidonic acid and the prostaglandin E2 series.

Infla-Menses

Bromelain was shown in a clinical trial to improve severe primary dysmenorrhoea, at least when applied to the cervix. All women in this study had instant relief of their pain, but don't try this at home – a buffer solution was needed, and you can get systemic relief when taking bromelain capsules on an empty stomach at the recommended dose. In another, 40 of 64 women found instant relief too, but it was ineffective for those with dysmenorrhoea caused by diseases like endometriosis.

Pomegranates

Pomegranates are a sweet, tart, juicy red fruit that have been popular for thousands of years. Not only do they taste good, but they also may help women with PCOS. A clinical trial of 92 women with the syndrome compared pomegranate juice alone, as part of a probiotic beverage, the probiotic beverage alone, and a placebo at doses of two litres per week (around 250-300mL every day). The women taking either the combined or probiotic-only treatment had improvements in insulin sensitivity, BMI, weight and waist circumference, as well as testosterone levels.

Pomegranates are rich in antioxidants, and so likely have anti-inflammatory effects on their own. However, they also contain a precursor to another beneficial compound, urolithin A, which requires certain intestinal bacteria to produce it. As explained by *LEAF Science*, the ellagitannins in pomegranates cannot become urolithin A without these bacteria. Its benefits lie in the ability to improve mitochondrial health (the cellular powerhouses), which contributes to us having happy, healthy cells that won't trigger inflammation. While research has shown antiaging benefits in older volunteers, it can be of use to you if you have been debilitated by illness (or you are older, and are reading this for your daughter or granddaughter). On its own, pomegranate extract is shown to boost mitochondrial function at select stages. The phytochemicals in pomegranates also affect the growth of probiotic bacteria and encourage production of the short-chain fatty acids that reduce inflammation, restore gut wall integrity and aid blood sugar control.

Cruciferous Vegetables

Cruciferous vegetables are part of the *Brassicaceae* family. They include broccoli, cabbage, kale and Brussels sprouts, and are a lesson in how foods don't have to be scarce to be special.

Sulphoraphane, found in cruciferous vegetables, is well-known for its hormone-balancing ability. However, lab studies found that it also has anti-inflammatory effects by lowering TNF-a, NF-kB, COX-2 and other mediators. Sulphoraphane may prevent inappropriate blood vessel formation, something fibroids trigger when they grow too big to be supported by existing ones. A population study helped to confirm this by showing that a higher risk of fibroids was tied to lower consumption of cabbage, Chinese cabbage and broccoli. In another lab study, the indole-3-carbinol (I3C) in cruciferous vegetables was suggested to help women with PCOS. Not only were hormones such as LH and insulin reduced, but certain inflammatory markers were too.

The best way to get the beneficial sulphur-containing compounds in broccoli is to sprout them! Sprouts are 20-50 times more potent than mature broccoli plants, and you can either buy sprouts or grow your own.

Infla-Menses

Moringa

Moringa (*Moringa oleifera*), or the "miracle tree", is gaining increased attention for its health benefits. My search engine, Ecosia, funds reforestation projects that often include it on their list of trees for its fast growth and economic benefits to local populations. The edible parts of moringa have strong anti-inflammatory properties, including effects on the COX-2 pathway and PGE2. You can find it as a tea, supplemental powder or dried leaf for use in cooking.

A study on the leaf extract showed that moringa halved PGE2, while another on a flower extract demonstrated its ability to cut both PGE2 and COX-2 by more than half. Moringa has also been found to boost production of our own antioxidants. When post-menopausal women were given seven grams of moringa leaves every day for three months, their levels of two key antioxidant enzymes rose by 10-18% while a marker of oxidative stress fell by 16%. Additionally, their levels of haemoglobin, the oxygen-carrying molecule on red blood cells, rose by 17%. This means it may help if you're anaemic. Besides its benefits for older women, remember that oestrogen falls during your period too, and may have some antioxidant ability.

What's more, moringa can be a great vegetarian source of protein and iron. 100 grams of dry leaf contains 29 grams of protein, and 25mg of iron. It's also high in magnesium, with an estimated content of 448mg per 100 grams; although you won't be eating this much at once, this is around the recommended intake. Like other sources of iron, boil the leaves first to remove antinutrients.

Don't write moringa off as a fad because of the "superfood" label. Foods with this label often are higher in certain nutrients and phytochemicals, and so can indeed have specific health benefits. They also increase the diversity of our diets and make healthy eating interesting by providing different flavours and opportunities to explore new cuisines. That new superfruit you just read about could lead you towards an amazing Latin American recipe, or inspire you to learn about native Australian bush food. Salad sandwiches get boring after a while.

Resveratrol

Red grapes, as well as peanuts and Japanese knotweed (used as a herbal remedy and in supplements) contain resveratrol, a well-known antioxidant. Sound familiar? It is the antioxidant well-known for giving red wine a "healthy" reputation. By reducing inflammation, it can help to discourage uterine cells from invasion, prevent overgrowth and reduce excessive blood vessel formation.

In clinical trials, resveratrol has relieved pain and lowered levels of an inflammatory marker linked with endometriosis. It may also help to modulate levels of oestrogen. An early lab study found that resveratrol can inhibit the F2-series prostaglandins that contribute to period pain in many women. It had a direct anti-spasmodic effect by preventing hormones, such as oxytocin, from causing uterine contractions. Oxytocin is not inflammatory itself, but can increase production of inflammatory prostaglandins.

In another lab study, resveratrol reduced the total area of adhesions by 80%, and their number by 60%. If you have PCOS instead, resveratrol can be effective in relieving metabolic syndrome-associated inflammation. It helps to regulate insulin secretion, the circadian rhythm and inflammation directly through NF-kB. These effects all use the SIRT1 gene, which may have broad antiaging, life-extending properties. A clinical trial in women with PCOS, where they took 800mg of resveratrol daily for 40 days, also found a benefit. There was a significant normalisation in the women's levels of testosterone, TSH (thyroid stimulating hormone), FSH and LH, while the levels of growth factors in their ovaries fell too. During an assisted reproduction procedure, they turned out to have more high-quality eggs and embryos.

Therapeutic doses of resveratrol can only be achieved by supplementation, especially because humans do not absorb it well. However, it doesn't hurt to eat red grapes and peanuts as a snack, especially if they're a substitute for chips and lollies.

Drink Your Tea

Tea, whether it is black, oolong, green or white, can be a great way to both keep your water intake up and inflammation down. While black tea has benefits of its own, green tea is more well-known for its antioxidant content. Both are from the same species, *Camellia sinensis*, but green tea is less oxidised. Matcha is the powdered form of green tea and is particularly high in an antioxidant known as epigallocatechin gallate (EGCG). This is a powerful inhibitor of excessive blood vessel growth, so it may make your flow lighter with regular consumption. It may also help prevent uterine cells from invading and attaching to other areas of the body.

For these reasons, research on endometriosis adhesions found that EGCG can reduce their growth. EGCG is another inhibitor of PGE2, partly through reducing COX-2 and oxytocin. This and other catechins in tea also lower production of arachidonic acid. Lab studies have shown that this is how it may reduce period pain, heavy flow and inappropriate growth of the uterine lining. Instead of cramping, it promotes a healthier pattern of contraction. And besides, tea is relaxing to the abdominal muscles anyway because of its warmth. Additionally, green tea extract at a dose of 800mg per day significantly reduced fibroid volume and symptom severity in a clinical trial, and improved quality of life compared to women in the placebo group.

The type of tea you drink matters in the case of primary period pain too. A population study of Chinese women found that black tea did not reduce the risk or severity of period pain, but oolong and green tea did. Oolong tea was linked with a 40% lower risk of mild pain and a 66% lower risk of moderate to severe cramping. Green tea had a similar effect, reducing mild period pain by 37% and moderate to severe pain by 58%. There was a possible link between drinking coffee or energy drinks with period pain, most likely because caffeine can increase muscle cramping. However, remember to only drink tea in moderation regardless of what type it is. Tea leaves are high in tannins, which bind to minerals like iron and prevent them from being absorbed. It's best to separate tea from meals.

Infla-Menses
Chocolate can be Healthy

Depending on how it is (or isn't) processed, chocolate can actually be another antioxidant, anti-inflammatory superstar! It is the most clichéd thing to eat during your period, but it turns out you have plenty of good reasons to enjoy it. The antioxidant effects of chocolate may even reduce insulin resistance, benefitting women with PCOS if it isn't too high in sugar. Research published in the *American Journal of Clinical Nutrition* shows that the flavanols in cocoa beans can lower insulin resistance by about one-third! It could provide a broad list of benefits for cardiovascular health by both reducing inflammation and increasing levels of HDL, the "good cholesterol". This is an area of concern in cases of PCOS.

The unnecessary amount of sugar and additives we see in the West do not have a place in traditional chocolate products. The Kuna people of the San Blas islands in Panama consume about three cups of a chocolate drink every day, with a total of 1880mg of procyanidins. This is the dominant antioxidant type in chocolate. Only 2.2% of Kuna islanders have high blood pressure, and their rates of diabetes, heart attack, stroke and certain cancers are lower than people on the mainland. People who do migrate to the mainland cities and adopt "modern" diets lose this protection. Their traditional diet also has twice as much fruit and four times the amount of fish as those in Panama City.

Why can chocolate have health benefits? First of all, chocolate could be more resistant to losing its antioxidant capacity than other foods. Some samples remain stable for at least 50 weeks, while cocoa beans and powder have even demonstrated stability after 75 years! It would typically take days or weeks for the antioxidants in other foods to degrade.

When you are making your own chocolate or choosing a healthier product than your average service station chocolate bar, it is important to know the difference between cocoa and cacao. Cacao beans, from the *Theobroma cacao* tree, are where all things chocolate come from. These are edible, but taste like a bitter form of chocolate. After being fermented and dried, beans are either heated at a low temperature and keep the cacao name, or at a high temperature and become cocoa. Cacao nibs are chopped up beans, cacao butter is the fatty part of the bean, and cacao powder is what you get when the fatty parts are removed and the rest is milled. The higher temperature destroys far more of the beans' antioxidant content, and Dutch processing degrades them even more.

Cacao powder has a reported ORAC rating (which measures antioxidant capacity) of 95,500, over triple that of cocoa powder at 26,600. Unfortunately, commercial cocoa preparations would often have no net benefit, due to added sugar, fillers and artificial ingredients. I recommend that chocolate be consumed as cacao, whether you buy the powder and make something at home, or purchase pre-made products (watch for sugar content).

Other constituents of cacao beans include oleic acid, also responsible for some of olive oil's properties, and stearic acid. Although it is a saturated fat, it isn't as bad as palmitic acid and is often considered "neutral". Dark chocolate (70-85% cacao) contains 36mg of magnesium per 100kcal, which is about 9% of the US RDA and three times the

Infla-Menses

amount of milk chocolate. Chocolate has a small amount of copper too, which we need traces of for sugar metabolism and the prevention of inflammation.

Anti-Inflammatory Fatty Acids

Some fatty acids aren't just used to build cell membranes and tissues. Certain types are turned into pro- or anti-inflammatory immune signalling molecules. For example, one signalling molecule is known as prostaglandin E1 (PGE1), which may protect against PMS by reducing the effects of the hormone prolactin. Many women with PMS seem to be over-sensitive to the effects of prolactin, and others have higher levels. PGE1 is made from gamma-linolenic acid (GLA), found in sources such as evening primrose oil. Magnesium, zinc, and vitamins C, B3 and B6 are needed to produce PGE1 too.

A study of 116 women found that a supplement containing GLA significantly relieved PMS, as measured by the PRISM scoring system. This is a calendar that lists 23 possible symptoms, each with a maximum score of 3, and is meant to be filled out every day of each cycle. Women given either one or two grams (1,000 or 2,000mg) of the supplement began with average scores of 27-29 before ovulation, and 98-99 afterwards until menstruation. At three months, these fell to 17-21 and 48-58 respectively; at six months, they dropped again to 8-9 and 28-35. The women taking the placebo only saw small, incidental drops in PMS scores. This was not linked to any change in hormones either, so the benefits of GLA were most likely caused by higher PGE1 levels.

The fats in fish oil – EPA and DHA – which the body can also produce from the essential fatty acid alpha-linolenic acid, may also be protective against menstrual problems. An early study from 1996 tested the effects of fish oil containing 1080mg of EPA and 720mg of DHA on women with issues such as period pain. When taking fish oil, they noticed significant relief in pain and other symptoms. Another from 1990 showed that a combination of evening primrose oil and EPA provided relief for 90% of the volunteers, who had endometriosis, compared to relief in only 10% of the women taking a placebo.

A more recent study tested the effects of fish oil on period pain in 172 young women at an Iranian university. Half took a 1,000mg fish oil capsule every day, while the others took ibuprofen as needed during their periods. Before the treatment started, two-thirds of women reported their pain as "moderate", and the rest described it as "severe". After one month, over 40% began to describe it as "low", and only one in six said it was still severe. At two months, one in four stopped experiencing any pain, and it was reported as low in almost half of the participants. Surprisingly, two months after stopping the fish oil, half of the women still reported no pain, and almost all the rest described only a low level of cramping – just 3% still said they had a moderate level of pain, and it was no longer severe in any treated volunteers.

If PMDD or general depression is a problem for you, you may benefit too. Omega-3 fats have been shown in population studies to lower the risk of serious clinical depression, measured by fish consumption. Many trials also find that omega-3 supplementation can reduce the severity of already-present depression. People with depression have, on average, lower levels of omega-3 fats, and lower levels are linked with greater severity of the illness. Students with lower omega-3 levels, or a higher omega-6:3 ratio, showed a greater inflammatory response to stress than those with more omega-3s or a better balance.

How does it work? Fish oil helps to relieve period pain by reducing the level of inflammatory prostaglandins, and was more effective than ibuprofen. Omega-3 fatty acids can also be made into chemicals called resolvins, which, as their name suggests, help to turn off the inflammatory response once it is no longer needed (i.e. after an infection or acute injury has been solved). On top of this, fatty acids can interact with certain genes that control inflammation, modifying how much they are expressed. For example, omega-3 fats reduce the expression of a gene that plays a key role in inflammation. The full benefits of improving our balance between omega-3 and -6 fats, whether through diet or supplements, can take some time. This is because the essential fatty acids are often stored in our cell membranes, which take three to four months to change over their fat content.

If you decide to supplement, I suggest a quality blend that reports EPA and DHA content on the label and uses an antioxidant like vitamin E to prevent the oils from going rancid. As for diet, I recommend a combination of fish and plant sources of omega-3 fats unless you are completely vegetarian. The average intake of EPA and DHA is very low, at least in the US, at only 0.08-0.16 grams per day! On the other hand, it takes around two servings per week of oily fish to provide you with an average daily intake of 400-500mg.

This amount is recommended after research has shown that it can lower the risk of cardiovascular problems later in life.

The best sources of EPA and DHA are herring, salmon, sardines, rainbow trout and white tuna. A three-ounce serving – around the size of a deck of cards – is enough for these to get you over one gram of EPA and DHA. As for plant sources of alpha-linolenic acid, flaxseed oil (7.3g/tablespoon), chia seeds (5.1g/ounce), hemp (22% of oil), walnuts (2.6g/ounce) and flaxseeds (1.6g/ounce) are the best. Only 21% of ALA is converted to EPA in healthy young women, and just under half of this becomes DHA. Men have a much lower conversion efficiency of 8% ALA to EPA. This means it is easier for women to become fully vegetarian or vegan without supplementation. Finally, when it comes to converting fatty acids to the anti-inflammatory prostaglandin E1 series, vitamin B3 provides necessary assistance. Some food sources of this are meat, wheat germ, peanuts, brown rice and buckwheat (no relation to wheat; it's gluten-free).

If you are vegetarian or vegan, hemp seeds are the best source of essential fatty acids. Hemp seed oil is roughly 80% unsaturated fatty acids, with the omega-3:omega-6 ratio sitting between 1:2 and 1:3; this is the optimal ratio for human health. It also contains vitamin E, terpenes and phytosterols, which are antioxidant and anti-inflammatory.

Don't worry about the omega-6 fatty acids if you have inflammatory issues; you don't need to overcompensate with omega-3s. A study of 100 patients with MS demonstrated that supplementation with evening primrose and hemp seed oil may help balance the immune system, so it is not excessively in favour of the inflammatory state. In this trial, the two oils also dramatically cut the relapse rate, and reduced MS disability scores from an average of 3.25 to 1.83 out of 10 (0 being no disability, 10 meaning death from MS). All of this demonstrates how powerful relieving inflammation can be, and that resolving brain inflammation may have strong effects on neurological or mental health complaints.

Probiotics and Fermented Foods

Probiotics, prebiotics and fermented foods help to optimise and restore the intestinal microbiome after illness, antibiotic use or years of poor diet. If you do need to take antibiotics, follow it with probiotics and prebiotics to ensure that the microbiome returns to a healthy state. Prebiotic foods, which feed gut bacteria, include onions, garlic, leeks, Jerusalem artichoke, dandelion greens and jicama. Consider it an opportunity – one of my patients noticed a reduction in the symptoms of her Asperger's Syndrome after antibiotics, and many people choose to reset the microbiome every year or two with a broad-spectrum herbal parasite cleanse.

Probiotics, found in both supplemental form and as part of fermented foods such as yoghurt, may help to reduce the inflammation which causes period pain. A clinical trial of 66 women with endometriosis tested three months of taking the probiotic species *Lactobacillus gasseri* against a placebo to see if it could relieve this condition and its extreme form of menstrual pain. After the three months, women on probiotics saw a 3.28-point decrease in pain scores (on a 10-point scale), from a start of 7.5/10. The placebo group saw a 2-point drop, but the treatment was still seen as significantly different. Both groups reported a decrease in pain using a descriptive 6-point score, which notes pain relief use and interference with work. The probiotic group experienced more relief here too, but it only became significant at three months when only they kept improving. As you can positively affect gut bacteria by eating enough vegetables and other plant foods, there may either be some placebo effect, or some women changed their diets (naughty when participating in a clinical trial, but understandable when you're in so much pain). This probiotic species produces immune chemicals that help instruct the white blood cells to remove out of bounds uterine cells. In endometriosis, they are less able to stop these from settling in other areas, and less able to remove inappropriate lining.

Research on probiotics has given us very inconsistent results over the years: some studies say they work, others don't. Besides how well we can maintain them through diet, another reason why introducing beneficial species has variable success rates is their resilience. Many common species that we introduce through probiotics as flagships, in order to start the shift to an anti-inflammatory/longevity-promoting microbiome, do not survive sitting on the shelf or digestion very well. Only a small percentage of them get to colonise the gut. There is an exception: *Bacillus coagulans*, the majority of which survives.

Bacillus coagulans is one of the very few known friendly species to form spores in difficult environments. They re-activate within a few hours after you eat them, and grow well compared to many other probiotics. This species was once thought to be part of the *Lactobacillus* genus, but had to be re-classified as *Lactobacillus* bacteria do not form spores. Why? Well, *B. coagulans* is another producer of lactic acid, which aids digestion and drives away microbes that are harmful or only okay in very small amounts. The form of lactic acid produced by *B. coagulans* is also the most effective (want the specific details? It's called the L+ optical isomer). You can find this species in probiotic supplements, as well as in some fermented foods, depending on the brand. In Australia, I found it in some brands of kombucha sold by supermarkets.

Several studies have shown that *B. coagulans* can help with conditions that often flare up at certain stages of the menstrual cycle. In an eight-week trial of the probiotic for patients with irritable bowel syndrome, only the treated group had improvements in pain and bloating. A small study involving people with Crohn's disease found a greater drop in disease activity and the rate of diarrhoea. Four out of five volunteers taking the probiotic were able to stop their anti-diarrhoeal medications, compared to one of six in the placebo group. As for arthritis, it significantly reduced inflammation, while improving mobility, pain and stiffness.

Don't want to take a pill, and prefer to use foods that both deliver and support friendly bacteria? One fermented food that can be very helpful for inflammation is kefir. The dominant species belong to the *Lactobacillus* genus, with documents like the Turkish Food Codex listing others such as *Acetobacter spp.* A study on 45 people with inflammatory bowel diseases found that drinking kefir for four weeks dramatically increased their intestinal populations of *Lactobacillus* bacteria, after some volunteers started off with almost none! Their levels of inflammatory markers fell, and in the last two weeks those with Crohn's disease had less bloating and greater general wellbeing.

Vinegar is another fermented food, that may act by improving blood sugar control and therefore indirectly relieving inflammation too. A pilot study of seven women with PCOS found that taking 15 grams of "apple vinegar" daily for three months significantly restored insulin sensitivity. This helped to rebalance their LH/FSH ratios, and four regained ovulatory menstrual cycles within 40 days!

Many naturopaths, myself included, encourage the use of apple cider vinegar (or a shot of lemon juice) for another reason. It improves digestion by stimulating the vagus nerve with its bitter flavour, so you produce more stomach acid, release more bile for fat digestion, and your digestive tract doesn't try to process food too fast. Stimulating the vagus nerve may also help us produce serotonin, and reduces inflammation by preventing the response to bacterial toxins from going into overdrive. Medical treatments working on this nerve have been used successfully for depression and inflammatory bowel diseases, but if you can maintain healthy vagus nerve function with a shot of apple cider vinegar, go for it! Just remember to embrace the bitter flavour – it's not the best taste in the world, but can be very helpful.

Finally, if you're dealing with long-term damage, broth is an important tool in healing the gut wall and microbiome, particularly in the early stages. If you eat meat, bone broth can be made from red meat, poultry or fish. Bone marrow and other connective tissues contain amino acids, such as glutamine and glycine, minerals and vitamins that the gut lining can use to knit itself back together. If you are vegetarian, you must combine plant sources of these nutrients. Cabbage (common), spinach and watercress contain considerable glycine, as well as sesame seeds and peanuts according to *SELF Nutrition Data*. Cabbage is also high in glutamic acid, which is a precursor to glutamine.

Antioxidants

Oxidative stress plays a key role in keeping the cycle of chronic inflammation going. You can see this in the case of sunburn, for example, where oxidative stress from too much sun exposure causes inflammation, which features pain, redness and swelling. This is because oxidative stress damages cells, so we need the inflammatory response to repair it, but even this will become harmful if prolonged by constant attack. Oxidative molecules are in turn released during inflammation, so a nasty cycle can result if there is no resolution. They are also a normal part of cellular energy production, usually made from oxygen, but while this is meant to stimulate production of our own antioxidants, this system can be overloaded by too many oxidants or not enough antioxidants and their building blocks.

Oxidative stress has been linked to the development and progression of endometriosis, as it is both a cause and effect of the chronic inflammation that encourages it to appear and take hold. When women with and without endometriosis were interviewed, those with the disease initially had a much lower intake of antioxidants than women who were healthy. Then for four months, half of the volunteers with endometriosis followed a high-antioxidant diet, which gave them high (but not excessive) amounts of vitamins A, C and E. They not only ended up with higher levels of these vitamins, but also more of their own antioxidants – typically stronger than those from food. One of our most important antioxidant enzymes, superoxide dismutase (SOD), increased by 40% after two months; another, glutathione peroxidase (often known as the master antioxidant), rose by 25% after three months. They're mouthfuls, but very important. The women also showed less markers for tissue damage. These markers indicate the level of oxidation of fats, an essential part of our tissues and what makes up almost all of our cell membranes. They may indicate or cause an increased size and number of adhesions outside of the uterus. As the women's levels of antioxidants rose, their inflammatory markers fell gradually and consistently over the four months.

You don't have to have endometriosis to benefit from vitamin E. Two studies on taking the vitamin for period pain found that a daily dose of 200IU or 500IU, from two days before menstruation until the first three days were over, significantly relieved period pain and made the flow lighter. It took two to four months for the women to see its full effects despite the intermittent use.

As for PMS, vitamin E can help relieve depression, anxiety and food cravings. Vitamin E works by acting as an antioxidant and partly blocking inflammation from the arachidonic acid pathway, including COX and LOX. It also helps to minimise unnecessary clotting. Its antioxidant ability is why some studies, including one during pregnancy, find that it is able to shrink fibroids. Fibroids are linked with low vitamin E through the resulting high lipid peroxidation. Just like EPA and DHA, only a small percentage of Americans meet the recommended intake for vitamin E, even though it's essential for protecting our fatty tissue from oxidative damage! Natural vitamin E from foods is more effective than synthetic vitamins because it stays around for longer.

Infla-Menses

It is vitamin E's ability to prevent prostaglandin production and arachidonic acid release that may also help it to prevent menstrual migraines. Studies have found it can reduce disability and the need for "rescue" medications too. Unlike pharmaceutical drugs, taking vitamin E at 400IU for five days during menstruation does not cause "breakthrough" headaches, where symptoms worsen once you stop treatment.

Vitamin C should accompany vitamin E in relieving menstrual migraines, as it can target neurogenic inflammation. This is where particular neuropeptides cause oxidative stress, and therefore tissue damage to blood vessels and other areas. You DO NOT want to let this continue! Complex Regional Pain Syndrome (CRPS), a debilitating chronic pain disorder, can result from inflammatory damage to the nervous system or other tissues. Thankfully, use of vitamin C at doses of 200-1500mg daily for about seven weeks following injuries is shown to significantly reduce CRPS risk. Migraines share the same root cause of oxidative stress and neuroinflammation, so vitamin C may help in these cases too. We could call migraines "CRPS of the brain".

Another ability of this vitamin may be lightening a heavy flow. In a small study of 18 women with menorrhagia, 16 of them found improvement when taking a supplement of vitamin C and bioflavonoids. These reduce excessive bleeding by making the capillaries stronger; damaged, weakened capillaries are often a result of inflammation and oxidative stress.

Consumption of many types of antioxidants is best, however; don't just rely on vitamin C or E-rich foods. This is because they regenerate each other in cycles, otherwise one molecule of an antioxidant could only stop one free radical each. For example, vitamin C regenerates vitamin E, while glutathione and vitamin B3 regenerate vitamin C. Food sources of vitamin E include nuts, seeds, butter, eggs, spinach, kale and sweet potato. It is best to consume vitamin E in whole foods. Hot-pressed oils, like palm oil, lose vitamin E during heat processing and can therefore damage your fatty tissue (and rainforests! Look up Ecosia's Indonesian projects to see some of the ways this is being addressed). Vitamin C is found in a wide range of fruits and vegetables, such as citrus fruits, berries and Australian native fruits like Kakadu plum and lilly pilly.

Spotlight: N-Acetyl Cysteine

N-acetyl cysteine (NAC) is a modified form of the amino acid cysteine, used in many supplements to boost liver health, as well as relieve oxidative stress by increasing production of the "master antioxidant", glutathione. Cysteine is the rate-limiting amino acid in glutathione; its levels control how much can be made. A 2013 study tested the benefits of NAC against endometriosis by assigning 92 women to either three months of supplementation at a dose of 600mg three times daily for three days each week, or placebo. Even though it was only one supplement, women taking NAC found that their endometriotic cysts shrank slightly, while the placebo group unfortunately had a significant increase in cyst size.

Infla-Menses

To be specific, the average cyst size among treated women shrank by 1.5mm, from 26.9 to 25.4mm, while it grew by 6.6mm if they were untreated. Eight cysts disappeared too, compared to four in the placebo group. Twenty-four (roughly half) of the women on NAC actually cancelled their next laparoscopic surgery! Only one non-treated woman cancelled hers. Additionally, period pain and chronic pelvic pain scores dropped by just over half. The researchers noted that NAC had more beneficial effects than standard hormonal treatment, so it may be a way out from having to suffer their often awful side effects. If you want to have a baby, NAC also doesn't affect fertility, and some women in this trial safely got pregnant.

NAC worked by reducing levels of the inflammatory COX-2, which increases the availability of oestrogen in the uterine lining. It does this by acting on prostaglandin E2, which is also the most powerful aromatase stimulant. Aromatase turns androgens – "male" hormones, such as testosterone; women have these in much smaller amounts – into oestrogens. This is one example of how cracking down on chronic inflammation can benefit the body in multiple ways, including hormone balance.

N-acetylcysteine can help women with PCOS by acting as a safe insulin sensitiser. When 100 women with the condition took either metformin or 1800mg of NAC every day for 24 weeks, their BMI, waist circumference and waist to hip ratio significantly improved. Fasting insulin and fasting glucose/insulin ratio also improved more, and so did their levels of free testosterone.

B vitamins

Low levels of vitamin B6, folate (B9) and/or B12, as well as poor folate metabolism, raise the level of homocysteine, which is meant to be only a temporary step in amino acid metabolism. Smoking and excessive caffeine consumption also raise homocysteine, while other nutrients that lower it are vitamins B2 and B3; betaine; choline; glycine and serine. High homocysteine causes oxidative stress and inflammatory consequences such as blood vessel dysfunction, platelet overactivation and cellular damage. Women with PCOS have higher levels of homocysteine, one reason why the syndrome carries a greater risk of cardiovascular problems. This is tied to insulin resistance.

High homocysteine can also result in menstrual migraine. Research on supplementing with vitamins B6, B9 and B12 has found a significant drop in both homocysteine and disability from migraine, and one has reported a drop from 60% to 30% in the prevalence of disability. This benefit is greater in patients with specific variations in the MTHFR gene, which is partly responsible for folate metabolism. If you are thinking of getting tested for your MTHFR status because of menstrual migraines or other PMS symptoms, don't hesitate! Just remember to research a reputable testing service that will protect your privacy.

Folate deficiency isn't just a problem if you're trying to conceive; it can contribute to depression too. A population study of over two thousand people found that low levels of folate are linked with higher depression scores, particularly in women. High total homocysteine or low B12 was not linked to depression except in older adults. Besides keeping homocysteine in check, folate plays essential roles in the production of the neurotransmitters serotonin, dopamine and noradrenaline.

Food sources of vitamin B6 include whole grains, walnuts, bananas, navy beans and salmon. Folate is found in citrus fruits; peanuts and other legumes; green vegetables, such as broccoli and spinach; and mushrooms. Alcohol inhibits the enzymes that allow for folate absorption, so avoiding it is best if you have a MTHFR mutation. Amusing name, serious implications.

Vitamin D

Vitamin D is a strong immune modulator, regulating almost every type of immune cell. This means it strengthens appropriate responses and damps down unnecessary inflammatory reactions. It also helps to regulate cell growth and differentiation, while preventing inappropriate growth of new blood vessels.

Vitamin D deficiency is unfortunately very common, especially in high-latitude areas after winter. It's very important that we make an effort to spend time outside in the sun, but not so much that you get burnt, of course. If you do live in a high-latitude area, aim to go outside regularly for as much of the year as possible. If you live at a lower latitude like me, consider which time you go out. I prefer to avoid midday in summer.

The properties of vitamin D are why moderate sun exposure could be essential to overall health and longevity. A Swedish study of over 29,000 women, aged between 25 and

64 at the beginning, found that women who avoided the sun had a lower life expectancy. Nonsmokers who stayed away from sun exposure had the same impairment of their longevity as smokers who spent the most time outside. This translated to a 0.6-2.1 year loss of life, and was mostly from improved cardiovascular health. However, this was a study of southern Swedish women, where the sunlight is weaker than in areas such as Australia or Thailand. Always consider the time of day, strength of UV light where you live, and your family heritage.

You don't even get to put off the seemingly never-ending list of consequences either, as vitamin D deficiency may cause period pain too. A clinical trial of 60 women with primary dysmenorrhoea and low vitamin D levels compared 50,000IU of the vitamin to a placebo, which was given every week for eight weeks. This is a very high dose; on average, it's like taking over 7,000IU per day! Usually, 1,000IU is prescribed to gradually restore levels in a safe, cost-effective way. After eight weeks, there was a significant drop in pain scores compared to the placebo group, which was maintained until at least one month after treatment ended (the end of the study period).

A similar trial, this time involving 897 young women, also tested 50,000IU of vitamin D given weekly for nine weeks. All of them had either PMS, period pain, both or neither. After the nine weeks, the rate of PMS fell from 14.9% to 4.8%, and period pain fell from 35.9% to 32.4%. The percentage of women with both complaints dropped from 32.7% to 25.7%. Vitamin D use was related to relief in several PMS symptoms, including a tendency to cry easily and backache.

Infla-Menses

If you only have PMS, then it's still worth checking your vitamin D levels. A review of clinical trials found that vitamin D supplementation can significantly relieve symptoms such as anxiety, which fell by nearly 60% in one of them. Many women with PMS are deficient in the vitamin, while a higher dietary intake is related to lower symptom severity. It's not the only trial to show that vitamin D can relieve anxiety and depression either. One involving women with type II diabetes reported a fall in anxiety scores from 12.31 to 9.15, and a fall in depression scores from 11.88 to 9.88. Their inflammation levels dropped too.

If your period pain comes from an illness like endometriosis, it may still help you. An investigation of data from the second Nurses' Health Study found that being in the top fifth for vitamin D levels was linked to a 24% lower rate of endometriosis, compared to the bottom fifth. The researchers explain that the vitamin balances out populations of certain immune cells (some promote inflammation, others reduce it) and puts the brakes on production of inflammatory signalling chemicals.

Additionally, population studies have found that women with low vitamin D are more likely to have fibroids, and this could explain why African-American women are at a higher risk for developing them. Darker skin means lower sensitivity to UV light; it may protect you from being burnt, but it also reduces your ability to make vitamin D. Besides its effects on the immune system, both healthy uterine cells and those from fibroids were found to have vitamin D receptors, meaning that it can act directly.

Minerals

Calcium and Magnesium: The Twin Minerals

We know that calcium is necessary for strong bones, with 99% of the 1-1.3 kilograms in our bodies used to harden them. However, one of its functions could also be to regulate inflammation and immunity. When 20 healthy people at risk of colon cancer were given vitamin D supplements alone, their expression of inflammatory genes skyrocketed. If they took calcium alongside it, this was modulated to a healthier expression pattern. This shows us the importance of overall optimal nutrition, not just relying on one nutrient as a cure-all. The researchers noted that another benefit of calcium is its ability to partly stop haeme from damaging the gut wall, because the participants all followed a standard Western diet.

Magnesium is both a muscle relaxant and anti-inflammatory, as it is a co-factor in an enzyme involved in anti-inflammatory prostaglandin pathways (PGE1). An open study of women with primary dysmenorrhoea tested the effects of magnesium pidolate, at a dose of 4.5 grams daily, from ten days before their periods started until the third day. Magnesium was not only effective in relieving dysmenorrhoea for these women, but for others who only took it from the day before their period started to the second day of their cycles. Pepitas, spinach, quinoa, Brazil nuts, almonds, cashews, dates and lima beans are some good sources of magnesium besides fermented dairy and fortified plant milks.

Cases of PMS and depression can benefit from magnesium too. One study found that taking magnesium during the second half of the menstrual cycle relieves mood-related symptoms of PMS. It also reduced pain from the second month of supplementation. As for "regular" depression, a trial on 126 volunteers tested the effects of taking 248mg of magnesium every day for six weeks. Results began to appear in as little as two weeks, registering significant improvements on recognised questionnaires for depression and anxiety. It didn't matter how severe their depression was, and their age or gender didn't affect the results either.

In the second Nurses' Health Study, higher intakes of calcium and magnesium were linked with lower risks of endometriosis. Women in the top fifth of dietary calcium intake were 21% less likely to be diagnosed when compared to the bottom fifth. Being in the second or top fifth of dietary magnesium consumption was linked to a 14-29% lower risk, with the strongest relationship among fertile women. Inflammation, among other causes, leads to disordered muscle contraction in the uterus and Fallopian tubes. Calcium and magnesium regulate muscle contraction together.

Zinc

Zinc can help to relive period pain through its use by the body as part of antioxidant enzymes and ability to reduce the inflammatory COX-2 enzyme. It could also work by regulating circulation. Zinc has been demonstrated to relieve angina and Raynaud's phenomenon, two conditions where muscle cramping results in the restriction of circulation and severe pain. Women with endometriosis may have higher zinc requirements and are often deficient. Even mildly low levels can dysregulate the immune system and allow endometrial cells to migrate and grow in the wrong places.

The effect of zinc on menstrual pain was discovered by serendipity. In 1982, women taking high-dose zinc gluconate lozenges as a remedy for the common cold were taken by surprise. Their periods began on schedule, but they had no cramping, bloating or other PMS symptoms that would normally appear! They even worried that they were pregnant, as the absence of symptoms was so unusual. Only the zinc-treated women noticed these benefits, not the women taking a calcium placebo. Since then, protocols where a dose of 30mg, 1-3 times daily was prescribed 1-4 days before menstruation have been tested, and are effective in preventing period pain. In other research where volunteers took around 30mg of zinc, they suffered no significant PMS, but symptoms did appear in women taking 15mg per day.

A later case series of five women describes the varying situations where zinc can help. One was a 17-year-old girl who previously suffered from severe period pain which often kept her home from school, and ibuprofen was ineffective. When she took two 30mg doses of zinc from the last four days before her period to the first day of bleeding, she didn't experience any cramping, had no warning symptoms before it began and got to attend school. Another case was that of a 49-year-old woman, who suffered from severe period pain, pelvic floor pain, heavy bleeding, bloating and a longer menstrual period of eight to nine days. Ibuprofen didn't work for her either, and neither did other treatments. She took 60mg of zinc twice a day for three to four days before her period started. With zinc, she no longer had to deal with period pain, pelvic floor pain, heavy bleeding or longer menstruation (bleeding time shortened to five days). She

Infla-Menses
was also less bloated and wasn't as bothered by salt
cravings.

Selenium
Selenium is a trace mineral, meaning you only need a
tiny amount in the microgram range. Its major sources are
Brazil nuts, walnuts, cashews, onions, grains, seafood and
organ meats. Mercury in seafood prevents its absorption,
another reason to priotise the SMASH fish. Selenium reduces
oxidative stress by helping to regenerate glutathione; even
the "master" antioxidant needs assistance.

Supplementation with selenium could help if you have
PCOS, including if you are trying to conceive. A trial involving
64 women compared taking a daily dose of 200 micrograms
(do not take more than this) to a placebo for eight weeks, so
see how they would benefit. Six times as many women
became pregnant compared to the placebo group – six
versus one – and over 40% found relief from alopecia
compared to less than 10%. Almost half had less acne, but
only one in eight women taking the placebo noticed this.
Women taking selenium also had significantly lower levels of
inflammatory markers, inappropriate body hair and DHEA,
which can turn into either "female" or "male" hormones.

Herbal Medicine

Herbal medicine is considered to be the original
medicine, although theoretical understanding and clinical
practice have improved almost constantly. A common
argument from "skeptics" is that herbal medicine cannot

possibly work since life expectancy was 20-30 everywhere in the world until the 19th century. However, this was caused by high extreme poverty; lack of indoor plumbing and electricity; and those with money having a tendency to swing the pendulum in the opposite direction, by eating too many rich foods and spending too much time inside doing sedentary activities as proof of how wealthy they were. This also ignores the explosion in scientific research on herbal medicine that began in the mid-2000s. A book from 1991 that I bought second-hand from my college's library only discusses traditional uses, but books published in the 2010s that acted as our official textbooks are full of scientific evidence, with larger numbers of herbs from around the world and uses for them.

Herbal anti-inflammatories do not have the side effects of pharmaceutical drugs, but some can clash with drugs, other natural remedies and certain medical conditions (for example, licorice may raise blood pressure). This is why professional advice is necessary if you need therapeutic doses of herbs. Some herbal medicines more commonly known for other properties are also anti-inflammatory. Black cohosh and wild yam are typically used for hormonal issues; calendula, chickweed, cramp bark, chamomile, lavender, marshmallow and meadowsweet are soothing and analgesic, for example. Horse chestnut, lady's mantle and witch hazel are astringent, while St John's Wort is used for depression and licorice is given for fatigue or to assist in treating burnout.

A number of herbal medicines have been adopted and adapted by different cultures, with devil's claw being one example. This is a southern African herb adopted by

Infla-Menses
European herbal medicine for inflammation in back pain,
arthritis and headache. In a pilot study for endometriosis, a
dose of 400mg, four times daily significantly reduced pain at
four weeks in half of the volunteers, and all women reported
better quality of life and fewer symptoms at eight weeks.

Some "herbal" medicines, such as French maritime pine
bark, come from trees instead of small plants. A study of 58
women with surgically diagnosed and treated endometriosis
compared an extract of French maritime pine bark to a
promoter of GnRH. The bark extract gradually relieved the
symptoms of their disease, without affecting oestrogen
levels. Even though the GnRH promoter reduced symptoms
faster, they had somewhat returned by six months after
stopping it. Both groups had a drop in CA-125 levels, which
is a marker of inflammation. Women with less severe disease
responded better than those with more advanced cases.
French maritime pine bark works by being a powerful
antioxidant and anti-inflammatory. This and devil's claw are
just used as medicines, but there are many more that you
can include in cooking or drink as teas.

Medicinal Culinary Herbs and Spices

Herbs and spices have been traded for centuries because
of their flavour and medicinal uses. When you use them
correctly and in their natural state (as opposed to artificial
flavours, and preferably organic), they can be amazing!
Those that can be beneficial for menstrual health include
chamomile, cinnamon, Damask rose, fennel, ginger and
turmeric.

Alexandra Preston

Chamomile

If your mother or grandmother tells you to drink chamomile tea when you feel cramps coming on, she's right. Its antioxidant, soothing constituents are able to significantly relieve inflammation, and preparations of the herb are approved in some areas for related digestive conditions. One of them, known as apigenin, is found in parsley too.

As an extract, chamomile can be effective in relieving emotional problems, such as anxiety and depression, associated with PMS. After 90 women living at university filled out forms describing PMS symptoms every day for two months, they were assigned to either 100mg of chamomile extract or a dose of mefenamic acid, both to be taken three times daily. Emotional symptoms fell by 30-33% in women taking chamomile extract but only dropped by around 11% in the mefenamic acid group. Both groups also saw a 10-13% decrease in the severity of mastalgia (sore, tender breasts).

Closely related to chamomile, feverfew has been used for menstrual problems for over two thousand years, as well as psoriasis, arthritis, headache and of course, fevers. It helps dampen the histamine response and prevent arachidonic acid from being turned into inflammatory prostaglandins. You can find it as a tea too.

Cinnamon

Not only does it taste great, but cinnamon (*Cinnamomum verum*) can be another effective remedy for period pain. In a clinical trial, 76 Iranian students took three capsules each day containing either 420mg of cinnamon or a starch that acted as a placebo. They tested its effects on pain, nausea, vomiting and heaviness, measured by number of saturated pads, over the first three days of their cycles. Even though the women only took cinnamon for the first three days, the results were significant. Three hours after starting treatment, their pain scores were 6.6/10, compared to 6.8 in the placebo group. However, after 24 hours it fell to 4.1 as opposed to 6.1/10, and by 72 hours it was only 1.8/10, instead of 4/10 like the placebo half.

Cinnamon also significantly cut the amount of time they were in pain too. At the two and three-day points, they only spent several hours of the day with cramping (eight and three hours, respectively), instead of most of the time. As for heaviness, they were far less likely to need four or more pads each day. They had less nausea, which resolved more rapidly, and were not as likely to vomit – 32 of 38 women had no episodes in the first 24 hours, compared to 26/38 in the placebo group.

Cinnamon was effective because of its anti-inflammatory, anti-spasmodic effects that act on the prostaglandin pathway. That's all good for pain, but why did they ask about vomiting? Well, the prostaglandins that cause period pain also stimulate excessive contractions in the digestive tract, which results in nausea and vomiting if their levels are high enough. If you decide to use cinnamon, remember that too much can be irritating, so keep to the recommended dose – this study used 2.5g per day – and don't use pure oil.

My professional "ancestors", who were often known as the Eclectic physicians, also used cinnamon for heavy menstruation. This was not for prevention. Instead, doses of cinnamon were given as often as every ten minutes, which may have averaged out to be higher than the 2.5g in the above study, in order to stop flooding while it was happening. Do not try this without professional advice.

That's not all cinnamon can be used for. It has been prescribed for many years to treat fibroids because of this ability to reduce menstrual flow. As part of the TCM formula *Cinnamon and Peony*, it was demonstrated to be effective by both traditional experience and in clinical trials. Or perhaps you are struggling with PCOS or Metabolic Syndrome. In that case, *Cinnamomum verum* has been found to reduce glycated blood cells by 2.6 units, lower waist circumference, and even resolve Metabolic Syndrome overall in a trial of 116 people with the condition. By the end of the study, 34.5% of treated volunteers no longer had it, compared to 5.2% of the placebo group.

When I was studying, one of my classmates learnt just how potent true cinnamon can be. She has type I diabetes, but had to reduce her dosage of insulin if she wanted to continue eating cinnamon with her oatmeal, which she used to help control her blood glucose levels. Using anything as an adjunct to insulin does call for professional help; my classmate could only get away with this because she was well into her naturopathy degree.

Damask Rose
Rosa damascena, or Damask rose, is used in perfumes, food and herbal medicine. It has pain-relieving and anti-inflammatory effects, inspiring a study involving 92 young women living on-campus at an Iranian university. All had moderate to severe period pain, but none had previous surgery and they were not using the contraceptive pill as

Infla-Menses

treatment. Researchers compared Damask rose fruit extract to an NSAID in relieving period pain over the first 48 hours of two cycles, using capsules that appeared identical. During both cycles, the fruit extract and NSAID were roughly equal in their benefits, but the Damask rose difference is that it does not cause gastrointestinal damage.

Fennel

Fennel (*Foeniculum vulgare*) comes from the same botanic family as carrots and celery. It is not only a herb and vegetable, but also an anti-spasm and anti-inflammatory remedy able to reduce uterine contractions caused by oxytocin and prostaglandin E2. In an Iranian study, 50 young women took either 30mg of fennel seed extract or placebo four times each day, for the first three days of their periods. Over five hours after taking the extract, their average pain level fell from 5.56/10 to 1.2/10; in the placebo group, it dropped from 6.44 to 3.2/10. It also resolved for the month more rapidly among the women taking fennel extract.

A second trial from the same country involved 68 women, all university students living on-campus, but compared fennel extract with vitamin E to ibuprofen. At most points in time after treatment, the combination of fennel and vitamin E was a little more effective than ibuprofen, and significantly more so within the first two hours. Ibuprofen is an NSAID, and as I wrote above, these can have negative effects on intestinal integrity.

Ginger

Ginger (*Zingiber officinalis*) root is not just a popular spice for cooking. Some of its constituents are anti-inflammatory, acting on the cyclo-oxygenase-2 (COX-2) and

5-lipoxygenase (5-LOX) pathways. In fact, ginger can turn down the expression of the gene that tells our bodies to make COX-2.

One clinical trial of 150 women found that ginger powder, at a dose of 250mg four times daily, was just as effective as pharmaceutical pain relief for menstrual cramps. Later in a review of studies, ginger was found to significantly relieve period pain. It was not taken for the entire month, just for the first three or four days of menstruation. All seven studies in this review came to the same conclusion that ginger is effective. When it was compared to another treatment, it was equal or superior. Ginger reduced both the severity and duration of period pain, and (where this was measured) scores on a Menstrual Distress Questionnaire.

A heavy flow can be just as annoying, if not worse, than period pain. In a study looking at the effects of ginger capsules, 92 high school girls took either this or a placebo for three months, and filled in a chart tracking blood loss. They didn't take it every day, just from the day before their periods started and for the first three days of bleeding. Before the treatment started, the girls lost an average of 113mL of menstrual blood, well over what is defined as menorrhagia. This fell to 71mL during the first month of ginger supplementation, and eventually to 53mL at three months. Ginger's prostaglandin-lowering effects were credited for the girls' relief, which it does by reducing COX-2.

Ginger can help with PMS too. A trial involving 66 women tested its effects when taken from seven days before menstruation started, until the first three days of bleeding were over. Five hundred milligrams of ginger per day

Infla-Menses
significantly relieved physical, emotional and mental symptoms of PMS, while the placebo did almost nothing. To be more specific, physical and "behavioural" symptoms were halved by three months, while mood-related symptoms were only one-third of their previous level. Besides its anti-inflammatory effects, ginger also helps to break up clots and relieve nausea, making it a helpful companion to cinnamon. Seek professional advice if you are on blood thinners or have a clotting disorder.

Medicinal Mushrooms

Medicinal mushrooms, many of which are used in cuisines around the world, can be powerful healers. When some of my neurological symptoms from gluten intolerance didn't just go away on their own, I started taking a powdered blend including reishi (*Ganoderma lucidum*) and lion's mane (*Hericium erinaceus*) every day. After a few weeks, I finally started to build strength in my forearms when I had previously been unable to, and my persistent balance problems started to improve! So what about published evidence?

First, let's look at lion's mane, a protein-rich mushroom described as tasting like lobster or prawns when cooked correctly. This mushroom stimulates nerve growth factor production, which may be helpful in depression, anxiety and other neurological disorders. In a study where 30 women ate biscuits containing either lion's mane or nothing special for four weeks, their depression and anxiety scores fell if they had the "active" biscuits. It may also have antioxidant, immune system-regulating and neuroprotective abilities.

Reishi is a powerful immune modulator and antioxidant, but may also help women with PCOS. When 19 medicinal mushrooms were tested, reishi had the strongest effects against the enzyme 5-alpha reductase. This turns testosterone into a more potent form, and so can contribute to symptoms such as male-pattern body hair or irregular menstruation.

The most well-known medicinal mushroom in the West is perhaps shiitake (*Lentinula edodes*), which you can find in many grocery shops. Besides being an ingredient for dishes such as soups, a study involving 52 people found that it can boost and rebalance immunity. Not only did they show a stronger response against infection, but inflammation was reduced and they had higher levels of a type of immune protein that protects the gut wall.

It would take a whole other book to discuss every medicinal mushroom and all their benefits, but let's finish with the first I learnt about, cordyceps (*Cordyceps sinensis*). This one has been used for centuries in China to boost energy and overall health, so could help you too if fatigue has been an issue. A small trial where volunteers took cordyceps extract for three months found that it significantly improved exercise performance, which is often impaired if you have a history of chronic health problems. Why miss out?

Turmeric

Turmeric (*Curcuma longa*) and curcumin, the most-researched phytochemical in the spice, isn't just something I recommend because it works for me. It has broad anti-inflammatory effects, including those against the COX and

Infla-Menses

LOX pathways, because it is an overall inhibitor of the arachidonic acid pathway. Some of its anti-inflammatory effects come from its antioxidant properties and ability to balance the immune system too. What's more, curcuminoids relax smooth muscle, helping to prevent the spasms that create period pain. Curcumin is potent but safe well past the necessary dose, however I still recommend that you see a professional for a consultation, especially if you are on medication. Many women who struggle with their periods because of blood clots welcome the anti-platelet effects of turmeric and curcumin, but this, like ginger, could be risky if you take blood thinners or have a clotting disorder.

Turmeric has been used traditionally in South Asia by systems such as Ayurveda to treat menstrual disorders and speed recovery after childbirth for many years. You don't necessarily require an expensive supplement, as its antioxidant properties are not degraded by some traditional recipes. One, known as golden milk, is described below under *Starter Recipes.* Traditional Chinese Medicine (TCM) physicians have prescribed the root and rhizome of several *Curcuma* species for centuries too, since at least 500 AD. The root has often been indicated for activating circulation and healing, while the rhizome is commonly prescribed to promote menstruation and prevent blood stasis.

One benefit of curcumin verified by modern research is that it may be an effective remedy for PMS. A clinical trial of 70 women compared the effects of two capsules of curcumin or a placebo for seven days before their periods until three days after it ended, for three consecutive cycles. The treated women got to experience a drop in PMS scores from an average of 102.06 to 42.47; in the placebo group it only fell from 106.06 to 91.6 points.

Curcumin may also help with heavy periods by turning down excessive blood vessel growth in the uterine lining, as well as reducing growth of the lining itself. This can be the case in both inappropriate growth, such as that seen in endometriosis, and normal lining. It was only when I began to control my inflammation levels that my own periods became lighter, and turmeric/curcumin supplementation has been the most effective intervention. This effect against overgrowth could translate to curcumin being another part of fibroid treatment. A laboratory study demonstrated that it stopped fibroid cells from dividing, essentially by killing them off, but did not have this effect on normal myometrial cells.

Preclinical work also shows how curcumin may work against endometriosis. In one, curcumin shrank lesions in mice with the disease by impairing the function of a pro-inflammatory gene, as well as an enzyme called matrix metalloprotease-3 (MMP-3; insert dad joke about MP3 players here). It also killed off endometriotic cells using more pathways to do so than a common anti-inflammatory drug. MMP-3 allows for cell migration, and so would contribute to the appearance of endometrial cells outside the uterus.

In a second study, curcumin was found to act against the growth of the lesions seen in endometriosis by inhibiting activity of an enzyme abbreviated as MMP-9. This also reduced levels of TNF-a, and resulted in the lesions shrinking. A third demonstrated that curcumin can reduce levels of oestrogen, with higher doses having larger effects. Eventually, this translated into smaller lesion sizes; while curcumin started to affect oestrogen at the 48 hour point, it was only at 96 hours that the unwanted tissue growth began to slow. There were no effects on normal endometrial cells.

Curcumin could even help if you have depression, whether or not it is tied to your menstrual cycle. A review of six studies found that it is significantly effective compared to a placebo, especially at higher doses or when you take it for a long time. You would likely have to take it for at least six weeks to see a clear benefit. The traditional blend of curcumin and piperine (turmeric and black pepper) was just as good as a new formulation designed to boost absorption, known as BCM-95. Besides its antioxidant and anti-inflammatory effects, curcumin could be antidepressant by helping to balance neurotransmitters and protecting our brain and nerve cells.

Traditional Chinese Herbs

Traditional Chinese Medicine (TCM) is a system of medicine that has existed and evolved over several thousand years. Through its own understanding of health and disease, many diagnostic patterns seen in women's health issues are related to inflammation. Alexandra Yates, a TCM practitioner in my area, explains:

"All pathologies of inflammation will have an element of pain or discomfort. Women's health is complicated, so we don't only focus on what causes inflammation. There are root pathologies underlying, unique to the individual, that are treated along with this symptomatology, like a root and branch. An underlying cause could be Kidney Yin/Yang deficiency, Liver Blood deficiency, or Qi and Blood deficiency, and so on. It's a wormhole!

Some main branch pathologies of inflammation are:

Damp-Heat: Heavy, long periods. Blood is thick and contains mucous. There is a strong odour with discharge, which can be yellow or brown and thick. There can be a diagnosis of thrush or candida. Women with this pathology often have a damp-heat diet of greasy take away food, excessive meat consumption, excessive alcohol and milky coffee.

Liver Fire: Here, there is pain in the genital/anal region, odorous discharge, and headaches or migraines mainly in the temples, eyes or side of the head. Women with this pattern are hot and sweaty, angry and confrontational. They can have a high libido and high testosterone levels in the blood. This is caused by too many spicy, hot greasy foods; excessive alcohol and milky coffee. A high appetite from the excess heat further fuels the fire.

Blood stagnation: There is a sharp fixed pain in the lower abdomen, painful periods or lower abdominal pain. Blood stagnation means blood clots. There can be tumours, benign or otherwise, such as fibroids and cysts. Women can also have a diagnosis of endometriosis.

Qi Stagnation: Features pain with periods in the general area of low back or abdomen. It is better for mild exercise, or worse in the morning but eases as you get moving.

Infla-Menses

Cold invasion in the uterus: Very common. There are tiny blood clots in the menstrual flow, and sharp period pain that is better for warmth. It is caused by swimming in cold water or having sex during the period, and generally allowing cold to penetrate the low back.

Damp-Cold: There is a thick white discharge that has a fishy odour and feels cold. You may have a diagnosis of bacterial vaginosis. Damp-Cold has similar symptoms to cold in the uterus, just with the added discharge. It can lead to missed periods. Causes include too many cold raw foods, including too many acai berry breakfasts, and too many sweet foods, including fruit.

The recurring themes are:

1. Diet: Avoid too many cold, raw foods or too much dairy. Also avoid too many hot and spicy or greasy foods, and limit alcohol or excessive meat consumption.

2. Lack of exercise and sedentary jobs creating stagnation in the lower abdomen leading to inflammation. Increased circulation makes it harder for damp to form.

3. Keep your lower back and abdomen covered and warm.

4. Stagnant emotions. Learn to express emotions as they come up. Don't sit and stew on issues as it creates stagnation and damp in the body. If you are angry all the time, find out why rather than continuing to fuel it by emotional eating."

Many Chinese medicinal herbs have made their way to the West, and chances are you have seen some in commercial supplements. Two, peony and rehmannia, have been used in TCM and Japanese medicine together for centuries in the treatment of menstrual problems. Research usually (correctly) tests them together, and they have demonstrated clotting inhibition and reductions in prostaglandin production. Licorice and dong quai are also anti-inflammatory, and are often prescribed with these two herbs. Yet another anti-inflammatory herb from TCM is hibiscus (*Hibiscus sabdariffa*), which, like licorice, you may find in herbal teas. Its antioxidant content can reduce the levels of COX-2 and PGE2, so it may help with period pain and PMS. The related *Hibiscus rosa-sinensis* is traditionally used in Bangladesh to relieve excessive menstrual flow.

Herbal formulas used in TCM work by many different mechanisms. They are designed with synergy in mind to produce the maximum benefit, not to find a one true silver bullet. For example, an analysis of *Siwu* decoction (literally: four things) found 16 components and 24 pathways known to help period pain. These act on immunity, inflammation, pain perception, muscle contractions and hormonal balance. The four ingredients are *Shu² Di⁴ Huang²* (rehmannia root steamed with water or alcohol), *Bai² Shao²* (white peony root), *Dang¹ Gui⁴* (Chinese Angelica root) and *Chuan¹ Xiong¹* (Szechuan lovage root).

Ayurvedic Medicine

Ayurveda is the ancient system of Indian medicine, and like the European system of naturopathy, it treats conditions based on a holistic perspective. Although individualised, people are categorised into three main *doshas*: *vata*, the thin, deficiency-prone type; *pitta*, the fiery, inflammation-prone type; and *kapha*, the type prone to sluggishness but favours tissue-building. *Dosha* classification depends on your

Infla-Menses

predominant type, as we all have a degree of each. Some people are a mix of these; for example your skin may have *kapha* traits but mentally you're *pitta*.

Period pain is called *Kashtartava* (ill or painful + menstruation), and is described as a symptom of Ayurvedic disease classifications. Gynaecological disorders typically require the *vata dosha* to be rebalanced first, then treatment of other imbalances can begin. Some cases of endometriosis are *vata*-dominant in the early stages, then become *kapha*-dominant, and involve all three *doshas* if they progress to extreme severity. Treatment of endometriosis not only involves rebalancing *vata* and *pitta*, but also strengthening *agni* (digestive fire) and clearing out *ama* (toxins, whether they be metabolic waste, natural or man-made).

Many recommendations are anti-inflammatory, for example to avoid smoking and alcohol; as well as ensure regular exercise. Walking, swimming, some types of yoga, tai chi and qi gong are good for balancing *vata*. Fresh fruit like plums, dark grapes and pomegranates are advised, along with leafy green vegetables and cooking with ginger. Additionally, dietary supplements including B6, B12 and vitamin E can be prescribed. Most Ayurvedic treatment plans involve traditional herbal formulas too, which often have a broad range of uses. Dale Bredesen recommends Triphala to people diagnosed or at risk of Alzheimer's, but you could benefit at any age! This is a blend of *amalaki, bibhitaki* and *haritaki*, which acts as tonic and remedy for inflammation. You can take it as a capsule, or tea in its powder form.

Besides turmeric, one of the most well-known Ayurvedic herbal remedies is frankincense (*Boswellia spp.*). In

Ayurveda, Indian frankincense is known for acting against *vata* disorders. Also known as *salai guggal* and many other names, it has been used for centuries to relieve inflammation. It works by blocking the production of leukotrienes, which is how it has so many uses for inflammatory conditions and has won over traditional physicians around the world. Frankincense does this by inhibiting 5-LOX, that nasty little stimulator of inappropriate blood vessel growth and tissue migration. Its resin is included in the supplement I take.

Frankincense may also help to relieve dysbiosis and oral infections, two causes of systemic inflammation. Its resin inhibits certain pathogenic bacteria and disrupts biofilms in some species. In another study, an acid in the resin was the most potent antibacterial compound against oral bacteria. In traditional Iranian medicine, frankincense has been used to treat inflammatory bowel diseases. A study on 350mg of gum resin taken three times daily found that over six weeks, it induced remission in 80% of patients with grade II and III ulcerative colitis. Gastrointestinal inflammation can be very common in women with endometriosis – I had a friend at school with both Crohn's disease and suspected endo.

Herbal remedies are typically prescribed as formulas in Ayurvedic medicine. A case series on seven women with uterine fibroids (a type of *Granthi*, or encapsulated growth) involved them taking three formulas: *Shigru Guggulu, Kanchanara Guggulu* and *Haridra Khanda*, to be chased down with milk. Their ingredients included myrrh, moringa, turmeric, ginger, cinnamon and black pepper. The women ranged in age from 20 to 47, and all saw their fibroids either shrink or resolve completely after seven weeks. One enjoyed a resolution after continuing her treatment for longer. With results like this, such a treatment plan needs further study, as long as it respects the principle of individualisation.

Optimising Your Endocannabinoid System

Hemp has perhaps the most interesting journey through history out of any herbal remedy. Demonised for decades, the discussion around cannabinoids has recently begun to change. Older readers may remember "Just Say No"-type slogans, which have since evolved into legalisation efforts, debates on what exactly should be allowed and research into the potential health benefits of cannabinoids. It turned out that we actually produce our own cannabinoids, and those from hemp work by interacting with them and their receptors. If I listed the countries and states where you could legally buy hemp extracts now, it would most likely become outdated fast, as high-CBD products lose their guilt-by-association reputation. Hemp's very 20th century poor reputation has been so pervasive, that until November 2017 it was not even legal to sell hemp seeds or their oil as food in Australia, even though they contain no cannabinoids! Fortunately for those of us who cannot access CBD products, there are even ways to work around this.

What is the Endocannabinoid System?

Every human has a system of cannabinoids and receptors for them, known as the endocannabinoid system (ECS). The two major cannabinoids our bodies produce are anandamide (AEA) and 2-AG. There are two main endocannabinoid receptors: CB1, in the brain, fat, liver, muscle and bone; and CB2, which mostly works with the immune system but may also be present in the central nervous system. Sometimes, our cannabinoids interact with other receptors. Cell receptors, and things that bind with them such as hormones or cannabinoids, are like tiny locks which activate or turn down biological processes once their "keys" unlock them. Different cell types have different receptors on their membranes.

The roles of the ECS include pain perception, inflammation, immune regulation, neural protection, neuroplasticity and metabolism. A deficiency in endocannabinoids may contribute to conditions such as IBS, fibromyalgia, migraine and psychological disorders. These are quite common in young women, who are often ignored because they "don't look sick", and are often affected by changes during the menstrual cycle. Levels of anandamide actually correlate with oestrogen levels throughout your cycle. If the drop in oestrogen, and therefore anandamide, bothers you during your period, it makes sense for you to boost its levels so you can keep feeling great throughout the month.

It sounds too good to be true, but the ECS has so many regulatory responsibilities, which is also why nature knows best when working with it. How do we know? Well, for example, a drug designed to treat obesity by inhibiting CB1 was withdrawn due to dangerous side effects, namely suicidal ideation. There is far too much suicide in the world as it is; let's give our bodies the tools they need to regulate the ECS instead of hammering one pathway.

What Makes a Hemp Extract?
Cannabidiol (CBD) is the major cannabinoid in industrial hemp (as in not the intoxicating strains), and is now highly

sought after for its potential health benefits. It has demonstrated anti-inflammatory, analgesic, anti-nausea, anti-anxiety and antioxidant effects, and may also help prevent unwanted migration of cells, such as that seen in endometriosis. Cannabichromene (CBC) can also be anti-inflammatory and analgesic, and so is cannabigerol (CBG), a cannabinoid with lipo-oxygenase blocking properties. There may actually be up to 100 cannabinoids, but most of them are present in very small amounts.

A full-spectrum hemp extract is not short on terpenoids, which are the primary category of phytochemical in essential oils and give plants their aroma. Interestingly, cannabinoids and terpenoids are produced in greater amounts when light exposure is high and soil fertility is low. Some terpenoids, such as linalool and myrcene, are unfortunately destroyed by irradiation, which is required for government medical programs in Canada and the Netherlands. You don't need to live in a country or state where it is legal to sell hemp extracts as herbal remedies or supplements to get the benefits of these terpenoids, however, as they are found in many essential oils.

One of the most common terpenoids, limonene, has been shown in lab and clinical studies to help relieve depression and anxiety. If you get these symptoms during or before menstruation, you may benefit from lemon or another citrus essential oil, which can be inhaled or used as a natural perfume. Beta-myrcene also comes from hops (*Humulus lupus*); it is used in herbal medicine to aid sleep and is anti-inflammatory by acting on the prostaglandin E2 series. Alpha-pinene, found in pine extracts and *Salvia spp.* (sage) essential oils, is anti-inflammatory via the PGE1 pathway and may boost memory.

The major terpenoid in hemp plants is beta-caryophyllene, also seen in copaiba balsam (*Copaifera officinalis*) and black pepper (*Piper nigrum*). It is anti-inflammatory by the PGE1 pathway; can protect the digestive tract lining, possibly why it was traditionally used for duodenal ulcers; and has even been shown to act on the CB2 cannabinoid receptor at certain doses. There is no risk of cannabis-like intoxication with beta-caryophyllene containing plants. While CBD has been used as an aid to quit nicotine smoking, a clinical trial on 48 people testing black pepper essential oil found that it significantly reduced cravings. The combination of beta-caryophyllene (CB2 receptor stimulant), myrcene (relaxant) and pinene (stimulant), a blend also seen in hemp, was likely behind this effect.

Other Ways to Work with the Endocannabinoid System
One way to use the endocannabinoid system without CBD-containing hemp products doesn't necessarily cost you anything. You may be familiar with the "runner's high", described as: a feeling of elation, happiness, harmony, inner peace, unity with nature, increased energy and a dampened pain sensation. The traditional hypothesis was that this is caused by our bodies producing our own opioids. However, the major chemical thought to be responsible, beta-endorphin, binds to a receptor known to cause respiratory suppression, constipation and pinpoint pupils – the side effects of opioid drugs, and why they can be so dangerous. They are not seen in athletes. Beta-endorphin is also very similar to a stress hormone elevated during exercise, so

detecting it is yet another issue. More recent research points to the endocannabinoids as the answer.

In a study of trained male athletes either running or cycling for 50 minutes at 70-80% of their maximum heart rate, researchers found a dramatic rise in blood plasma levels of AEA. Part of this effect may be from running being a weight-bearing, pavement (or grass) pounding activity, as well as a repetitive movement. I would recommend moderate activity if you have serious menstrual issues, and do not have the energy for much more than a walk or jog.

Repetitive movements that don't require much thinking are more likely to activate the right areas of the brain to produce cannabinoids. In fact, multiple studies of trained athletes involving hiking at high altitudes, running and cycling all saw significant AEA boosts, sometimes during recovery too. Beta-endorphins did not rise until they reached 75% maximum output (and fell during recovery!), poking another hole in the opioid theory. Swimming is another repetitive-motion exercise that can increase endocannabinoid production, especially if you're doing it in cold water. Exposure to the cold is known to boost levels of endocannabinoids and raise the density of neurons positive for CB1 receptors. However, you do have to find a form of physical activity that you enjoy, as forced exercise is interpreted by your body as STRESS! It won't increase endocannabinoid levels, and is more likely to reduce CB1 signalling.

But why cannabinoids? First of all, the pain-relieving effects of AEA may be called on to help us get to whatever the finish line may be. From an evolutionary point of view, this could be a predator, so stopping because of discomfort could be dangerous. Low doses of cannabinoids are still enough to relieve chemical-induced pain, such as what you get from lactic acid build-up. AEA also inhibits inflammation and swelling, reducing the damaging effects of vigorous exercise and allowing for a beneficial, tissue-building response later. The relief of stress and anxiety may be a positive side effect, or could be a way to help us think clearer if we are escaping a threat. Another effect of exercise and AEA is that it opens up the blood vessels, thus boosting circulation, and opens up the airways so we can get more oxygen in. Better circulation can help with removal of toxins and inflammatory mediators, as well as nutrient delivery. Overall, this research shows that walking, jogging, running or cycling may be helpful in relieving mild to moderate cramping and the emotional symptoms of PMS.

Apart from exercise, how else can we work with the endocannabinoid system to relieve inflammation? To start, we have to ensure a sufficient intake and balance of "healthy" fats, including essential fatty acids. One reason why we need some omega-6 fats is that arachidonic acid is needed to produce AEA and 2-AG, but too much will lead to an excess of these and a desensitised EC receptor system. This can, among other things, overstimulate appetite. Olive oil is rich in fatty acids such as oleic acid (non-essential, but has benefits), upregulates the CB1 receptors, and is much healthier than canola and other vegetable oils because of its antioxidant content.

An overall deficiency in EFAs can reduce EC production, and even just supplementing with EPA and DHA can increase ECs in this situation. Omega-3 fatty acids may also increase the number of EC receptors, as well as other fatty acid-derived substances our bodies produce to assist our ECs. A deficiency of omega-3 fats, which is unfortunately very common, may stop the ECS from working in the brain. What about when the ECS is overactive, such as in obesity? Krill oil can reduce EC levels in obese people, but not in those with a normal weight. As omega-3 fats are needed for ECS signalling, it's safe to assume they regulate the system, instead of switching part of it on or off.

Eat your vegetables, too. Diindolylmethane (DIM) is found in cruciferous vegetables such as broccoli, kale, cabbage, cauliflower and Brussels sprouts. You may have heard of DIM because of its disease-preventing, oestrogen-clearing properties often promoted to women with menstrual problems or a high risk of certain illnesses. Besides helping oestrogen metabolism, DIM also has anti-inflammatory effects through the ECS, by binding to CB2 receptors. This can therefore help if you have both hormonal and inflammatory issues underlying difficult menstruation. Some people like to grow their own broccoli or watercress sprouts, which have higher levels of DIM and related compounds. You can find kits in some health food stores or DIY instructions online. Growing your own sprouts is often cheaper than supplementation.

In recent years, we have learnt that other herbs and supplements completely unrelated to hemp affect the ECS too. Many anti-inflammatory herbs and nutrients may partly work by acting on the ECS, as inhibiting COX-2 blocks conversion of AEA and 2-AG into other substances. The popular herbal remedy echinacea could stimulate the ECS without causing a high (it's pronounced ek-in-ay-sha; I had a teacher who first thought it was "e-chin-a-see-a" because she studied online). Some of its phytochemicals can bind to CB2, which is one way that it modulates the immune system. Others prevent AEA breakdown. As they only significantly affect CB2, echinacea is not intoxicating. *Ruta graveolens* and noni fruit (*Morinda citrifolia*) also have weak affinities for CB2. Flavonoids from red clover (*Trifolium pratense*), soy, tea and other plants can somewhat slow the breakdown of our cannabinoids, increasing their levels in the body. EGC-3-O-gallate from green tea also binds to CB1. Although curcumin can't bind to CB1 receptors, it raises EC and nerve growth factor (NGF) levels in a way that is dependent on these receptors. Copal incense, from *Protium spp.* (this is in the same botanical family as frankincense), contains a phytochemical with a high affinity for both CB1 and CB2 receptors. Finally, *Lactobacillus acidophilus* has been shown to increase CB2 production in lab studies where they were grown with human intestinal lining cells.

You don't have to be "good" all the time, either! Certain so-called "vices" or luxuries may provide health benefits via the ECS too. Interestingly, this includes part of caffeine's effects. Caffeine may increase the activation of CB1 receptors by cannabinoids, and prevent their downregulation by "social defeat stress" (think slipping up during public speaking or letting a bully's – ah, bull – get to you). However, whole, natural coffee is far better than caffeine alone, so stay natural and unprocessed instead of sugary energy drinks. Chocolate may work its magic through the ECS too by slowing the breakdown of anandamide, as well as by raising BDNF levels (this is important if PMS affects your mental health). Some research suggests that cacao or cocoa could contain anandamide, but they have inconsistent

Infla-Menses

results. Although expensive, black truffles do have anandamide.

Alcohol, however, does not help your ECS. A human trial comparing wine, grape juice and water found that blood levels of ECs drop within 10 minutes of drinking alcohol. This wasn't much, either – only a 250mL glass of wine! Chronic alcohol abuse can impair ECS function by desensitising receptors and downregulating their production. Receptors on cells get recycled and reproduced all the time, so it is possible to help or harm the ECS on a daily basis. A desensitised receptor functions less, while a downregulated one won't work at all. Some manmade toxins can negatively affect ECS function too. Pesticides such as chlorpyrifos and diazinon alter normal signalling, and piperonyl butoxide, a synergist added to some insecticides (e.g. pyrethrum), reduces CB1 activity. Phthalates may block CB1 receptors too. Watch out for plastic water bottles and food packaging!

Lifestyle, Energy and Mindset

Emotional Freedom Technique (EFT)

Emotional Freedom Technique (EFT) is like a hybrid between energy medicine and counselling, although you do not have to be a counsellor or acupuncturist to practice it. So what exactly does it involve? EFT combines tapping on a series of acupressure points with talking about the issue as a safe form of exposure, and then adding statements of self-acceptance. As a result, you can tap on the problems yourself anywhere, any time after a consultation. I and many other practitioners have successfully used it to help clients overcome unhealthy lifestyle habits such as smoking, alcohol over-consumption and poor dietary choices; traumatic memories and more. One reason why it works is that stimulation of the specific meridian points dampens overactive responses by the amygdala, a part of the brain responsible for negative emotions like fear and anger.

Let's start with smoking - so why use EFT to kick the toxic habit? It is no secret that conventional, reductionistic and sometimes quite patronising methods to help clients quit are often failures. Ninety-five percent of attempts at quitting are unsuccessful within a year, and there is still a risk of relapse afterwards. Success depends on experiences during the quitting and post-quitting phase, and how well interventions deal with the "benefits" of smoking.

Emotional Freedom Technique can directly address two of the biggest causes of sustained cigarette use: their function as a "tranquiliser" and withdrawal symptoms. Smoking is a common and once-accepted way of relaxation, of avoiding negative feelings. Withdrawal symptoms are typically emotional, such as anxiety and irritability, and can be worsened by the fear of experiencing them. Many people even think they mean that their body "needs" cigarettes! The therapeutic relationship with an EFT practitioner can help to deal with the other underlying cause, which is the powerful mental associations we can make between cigarettes and situations such as meeting with friends who smoke, stressful times or a favourite drink.

The issues to be talked about and tapped on typically fall into two categories: what are the downsides to quitting, and what are the advantages of remaining a smoker? Some reported "downsides" include fear of losing friends; fear of weight gain and fear of losing part of one's identity. Even "If I quit, I will have to achieve more" has been reported by clients in Peta Stapleton's study! When it came to perceived advantages, statements included "I will remain thin", "I can be like my father" and "I can get away from people". The graphic warning labels that cover cigarette packaging in Australia, and even the photo of a bird feeding their baby a cigarette filter – which has gone viral at the time of writing, mid-2019 – may shock people, but do not address why someone smokes. I even know nurses who used to smoke, despite seeing people die from the illnesses cigarettes cause, because it was an accepted way of being allowed outside for a break.

When using EFT, the exact words we tie to a situation or feeling are essential. For one client in an Australian study, tapping on "Even though I want this smoke, but I don't" had no effect. However, tapping on "Even though I have this habit and don't want to have this habit anymore" was effective in three rounds. This same client found that underneath this were feelings of self-consciousness, lack of goals in life and inadequacy in relationships. One month later, he found tobacco products too revolting even for special occasions and was more confident when asking to take breaks at work.

Poor dietary habits, such as food and alcohol cravings, are much more socially acceptable than smoking but can be just as harmful. We're told that we need junk food and alcohol to "enjoy life"; that it's "better to be fat and happy than skinny and miserable", even though only *some* people have a naturally larger frame; and that alcohol must be okay because of the link between moderate wine consumption and longevity in *some areas* (although grapes from those Blue Zone regions grow in particularly high-quality soil). Someone (not a client) even said to me that she'd "rather die happy" than improve her sugary diet – but isn't that an oxymoron?

Fortunately for those who are overweight or obese from overeating, EFT is also effective for preventing inappropriate cravings. Overeating is commonly caused by low serotonin, in order to correct the deficiency; negative emotions such as anger; and learned responses to situations. Once again, strategies like removing offending foods from home often don't work because they ignore why people eat them.

In another study led by Peta Stapleton, 96 overweight and obese volunteers with severe food cravings signed up for a four-week EFT program. Their craving severity and multiple measurements of self-control, as well as body weight and body mass index (BMI) were assessed from the beginning until one year after treatment ended. They had lost an average of 5.05 kilograms, or 11.1 pounds, by the one year-point; and they did not see their cravings return or substitute them for another food. The example case described in detail was that of MH, a 49 year old man who worked in telecommunications. He chose to focus on carbohydrate cravings, specifically pizza and peanut butter on bread, which he rated at a severity of 9/10. After several rounds of tapping, his craving severity dropped to 3 out of 10. When he returned to eating pizza and peanut butter, he only enjoyed them on occasions and didn't feel a compulsive need to have them. He and other participants then used EFT in their own time for other issues, including alcohol addiction. Some of the emotions surrounding food were guilt over throwing food away, fear of change and a sense of obligation to stay the same for others.

We now know that mental and emotional issues can affect the balance of the immune system, as well as countless other pathways in other areas of the body. This is especially the case in PTSD, where sufferers are in a constant fight-or-flight state; the debilitating nature of this disorder has led to many trials testing EFT for various types of trauma. When a small study of 16 veterans compared a course of ten hour-long EFT sessions to usual treatment, they not only measured changes to their PTSD scores, but also the expression of 93 different genes. Their PTSD scores fell by an average of 53% over the ten sessions and their expression of six genes changed significantly. These genes are involved in regulating inflammation and the immune response, but are known to be affected by stress. The saying that "it's all in the genes" is so often misused, because it isn't just about what we inherit from our parents. It's also about whether those genes are turned on or off, and by how much. You can see it in all the different types of cells in our bodies, which all have the same DNA, or in people who are closely related but have very different health statuses. Other markers of psychological health measured by this study showed significant improvements too: pain, anxiety, depression, phobic anxiety, insomnia, obsessive-compulsive behaviour, hostility, paranoia, psychoticism and interpersonal sensitivity. The benefits of EFT even persisted until at least six months after the treatment course ended, so there were likely long-term benefits to the veteran's thought processes.

Energy Healing

Misunderstood and underrated, energy healing may help to resolve a range of physical and psychological complaints, including inflammation. You may think it is just a placebo, but a study on mung beans (*Vigna radiata*) tested the effect of a standardised shamanistic growth and development ritual, performed by a Swiss spiritual healer. The experiment was conducted twice, on 84 treated seeds and 84 controls each time, and those that received energy work grew more than the controls. On day seven, they were 26% longer, with a stronger effect size at the germination pot level (high) than the seedling level (medium). Another study from *The American Journal of Chinese Medicine* had similar results. Here, energy work was found to modulate gene expression in order to dramatically speed germination. This is important because seeds cannot be influenced by the placebo effect. They cannot simply want to think they are growing faster, nor can they doubt the effects of energy work.

In humans, energy healing is no joke either. There have even been peer-reviewed studies showing that it can be effective. Let's look at reiki as an example, because it is one of the most common forms. A review of 13 studies, all involving over 20 participants each, found that eight demonstrated reiki to be effective. Four did not, but were of poorer quality, and one clearly showed inefficacy.

Much of reiki's effect seems to be via the parasympathetic nervous system. For example, one on burnout syndrome showed improvements in the two important markers of heart rate variability and body temperature control. Another on 120 people with various chronic illnesses showed that reiki improved pain, depression and anxiety more than placebo, rest or muscle relaxation techniques.

The only study that did not show any effect was on patients with fibromyalgia. According to *The Body is the Barometer of the Soul,* the overall "theme" with muscles is guilt, and communication in the case of nerves. As for menstrual issues, there are often themes of competing for outside love as a substitute for self-love, fear of living (PMS) or a need for spiritual growth. These require something where you can talk about the underlying emotional issues, only receiving healing energy is not always sufficient.

How far can it go? In a review of reconnective healing, another form of energy healing, a case study on a 74-year-old patient with emaciated legs was described. He was unable to walk without a walker for six months prior to his healing, and received three 45-minute reconnective healing sessions from a level III practitioner while lying on a massage table. The effect of reconnective healing was analysed by measuring electrodermal activity (EDA), with an apparatus for median identification (AMI). What this means is that the device measures electroconductivity in the body. After healing sessions, this displayed significant changes, which may have been partially caused by altered circulation and sweating. At the end of the third session, the EDA was 60% larger in the legs was 60% greater than in their upper body, indicating more sympathetic nervous activity. When EDA before the total healing period was compared to that afterwards, it increased by 49% in their lower body and dropped by 22% in the upper body. This means that blood flow was re-distributed from the upper to the lower body. Right after the third healing session, the patient decided to stand up without help and walk without their walker.

Additionally, a small trial comparing reconnective healing, reiki, physical therapy and sham treatment on shoulder pain found that reconnective healing increased range of motion by 26 degrees, and reduced pain by 24%. Reiki, physical therapy and rest only increased range of motion by 20, 12 and three degrees respectively. Perhaps the most surprising result I could find was an instance where a woman, who previously had three strokes, regained her ability to walk without her walker after traditional indigenous Australian energy healing. It surprised me the most because it was actually reported by a mainstream news outlet.

I am not trained in reiki, but instead with Diamond energy healing. I was one of the first through the Diamond Matrix Masters course. We rely on alignment with all parts of ourselves, our own decrees and our intentions of where to impart the Diamond energy, unlike reiki where specific symbols are used. I finally resolved my TMJ dysfunction with Diamond energy healing, after years of it appearing, trying different therapies, then it going away for a while. The

Infla-Menses

caused seemed to be an energetic holding pattern, subconsciously created and lodged in my mouth, from an unknown source (for example, a belief or negative event). It resolved overnight, even though previous attempts with other therapies took months to reach similar results. To make things better, the issue never returned and I was able to enjoy pomegranates for the first time in years! The self-mastery parts of this course help with, among other things, prevention of these issues reappearing.

My friend Kageni Njeru, also an energy healer, explains that "Cells are constantly communicating with each other, and the DNA is identical in all cells. There is constant communication." In fact, she once knew a woman who died at 55 after believing such a short life ran in her family. "Your cells listen to what you say and think."

"Your cells replicate. You get a new skin every month, but how many people DON'T say "I want you to look younger", I want you to look healthier"... but your cells are you! They have your name on it! When it replicates, we have the power to instruct our bodies! We are the masters of our own bodies, our spirits, until we give someone else the power to dictate that for us."

As a shaman, she says, "We have a way of asking questions; the root cause can be on any level. For example, a physical illness could have been from fighting over land with their brother – stress caused it. We ask, 'What is the thing causing this issue'; it could even be related to past lives or ancestors."

Alexandra Preston

In my own experiences with energy healing, I have noticed the same thing. To help a friend speed up their healing from an injury, I had to identify emotional causes (lack of self-care was one) and teach them to withdraw their energy exchange from the experience. Secondary gains were another major issue. In the case of menstruation, one that I often see in the holistic health world is that pain and fatigue have the "benefit" of giving us time off to spoil ourselves or be spoilt. What about flipping this story? You *deserve* to be spoilt anyway during menstruation because of its life-giving associations; as I wrote above, the "blood" contains stem cells which could provide many with complete, rapid healing.

I also had to remove the belief that we "need" injuries, illness or loss in order to learn "life lessons". We are adults, not children who need punishment. We can instead learn and challenge ourselves with joyous creations: perhaps hiking, learning a new sport or art form, or even joining a public speaking group will help you with personal growth. Hey, even a bad date or last-minute, unwanted list of errands to run for someone is better than a health problem!

Besides, multiple spiritual schools of thought state that a new era is emerging, where we are about to reclaim our power as masters. Some say that this has been unfolding since 2012; others say that the full force of the new energies will appear by 2029. Many "lessons" learnt from health problems and all their pain and limitations would therefore become irrelevant. I like to compare them to a kerosene lamp: they may provide some enLIGHTenment, but they are harmful just as kerosene damages human and environmental health. Lessons from an interesting challenge are like solar

Infla-Menses

lamps with attached USB phone chargers: superior lighting with side benefits instead of toxic effects.

Homeopathy

While not solely working on inflammation, homeopathy can be a very effective tool in relieving menstrual complaints. Homeopathy is a system of natural medicine founded by Dr Samuel Hahnemann in late 18th century Germany. It uses diluted solutions of a vast range of substances, which are potentised by succussion (banging it against your hand or using a machine to shake it in this way).

Although skeptics are quick to mock homeopathy for the use of dilutions, quantum physics has begun to develop explanations of how it works. This is a highly specialised field, not something your average surgeon or allopathic nurse would study in-depth; just look at the terms used in the next two sentences. Using quantum electrodynamics (QED) principles, it is argued that the dilution/succussion process creates conditions for something called "coherence domains" to appear in the water. These code the original substance's information (as phase oscillations) and can transfer it to a living organism. Disease, however, occurs when the multi-level coherence of the human (or animal) body is disrupted.

How does all of this benefit you? For example, homeopathy may be effective for endometriosis. A study of 50 women with deeply-infiltrating endometriosis tested homeopathic oestrogen, in what is known as a homochord of three potencies, against a placebo over 24 weeks. Five aspects of chronic pelvic pain were collectively measured as

Alexandra Preston
the primary outcome, but quality of life and depression were also taken into account. The average pelvic pain score, with a maximum rating of 50, fell by 12.82 points in the homeopathic group. Dysmenorrhoea, non-cyclic pelvic pain and cyclic bowel pain were relieved the most, but there was no significant relief seen in the placebo group. Mental health and vitality also improved in those taking homeopathic oestrogen. The women in this study were taking their remedy (or placebo) every day for 24 weeks, while in acute homeopathic treatment, you have to stop when symptoms improve. It is a highly individualised therapy, so you must seek professional guidance.

A study from Jerusalem involving 103 women with PMS was designed in a more individualised manner. Only those whose symptoms matched one of 14 pre-selected homeopathic remedies were included, but were assigned to either their remedy or a placebo. Most symptoms in each cluster are what we would normally consider part of PMS, while a few were "unusual" such as a craving for soft eggs or a tendency towards jealousy. I learnt to differentiate between remedies by seemingly strange symptoms and personality traits. With homeopathic treatment, the women had lower overall PMS scores, needed 75% less medication and took 91% fewer sick days. Some remedies seemed to be more effective than others. Women in the placebo group experienced less relief, only reduced medication by 36% and did not take fewer sick days. General health improved too. Outside the premenstrual phase, women taking homeopathic medicines had 74% fewer days off sick! The benefits of homeopathy may have still been underestimated, however. Remedies are given again if there is any recurrence of the symptoms, and often the remedies are changed as symptoms lift and a new pattern emerges. Homeopathy was still deemed as overall effective.

Low-Level Laser Therapy (LLLT) and PEMF

Besides hemp and the endocannabinoid system, the other relatively new development that looks like it will define 21st century healthcare is regenerative medicine. This isn't just about stem cell therapy. Treatments such as low level laser therapy (LLLT) and pulsed electromagnetic field therapy (PEMF) are also growing in popularity, whether patients have serious degeneration and injury ... or you just have menstrual problems.

An Egyptian study of 50 university-age women with dysmenorrhoea compared the effects of PEMF and LLLT on both reported pain and prostaglandin levels. PEMF involves an electrical energy, and generates magnetic pulses through the tissues. These trigger electrical signals that relieve inflammation and pain, aid range of motion and encourage cellular repair. It is used as an anti-inflammatory, to enhance wound healing and to stimulate neural regeneration. LLLT involves a "cold" laser emitting red or infrared light. It is an anti-inflammatory and analgesic, and can influence serotonin metabolism.

For this study, all women were treated on the first and second day of menstruation. They were given their assigned treatment in the pelvic or most painful area and over the L4-S3 spinal nerves. Prostaglandin levels fell from 76.01 to 61.79 in the PEMF group, and from 74.98 to 65.68 in the LLLT group. Their differences between each other weren't seen as caused by the treatment, so both therapies were deemed roughly equal in biochemical efficacy. However, pain levels fell more in the PEMF group, from 3/10 to zero, as opposed to 3/10 to 2/10 in women receiving LLLT.

Interest in PEMF is not new. An early case series from 1994 documented "unusually effective and long-lasting" relief from pelvic pain caused by various health conditions. These included period pain, endometriosis and ruptured ovarian cysts. Sixteen patients representing 18 episodes of pain got to experience marked or dramatic relief, while another two patients (representing two episodes) had some incomplete relief.

They might sound easy, but frequency settings matter! PEMF used 50Hz frequency and 60G intensity, while LLLT used a setting of 904nm. Professional training is necessary – it's not just waving a machine over the patient's body. Some specific wavelengths will help tissue heal, but a slightly different one won't. *The Brain's Way of Healing* reveals to us the effects of correctly using LLLT: cartilage regeneration in arthritis; serious wounds closing up; and of course, traumatic brain injuries being healed over months of regular treatment. The frequencies mentioned in this chapter, by the way, are 660nm (red) and 840nm (infrared).

How does it work? Some frequencies can resolve the inflammatory process, boost circulation and improve cellular energy production. There is a light-sensitive molecule in our mitochondria, the parts of the cell where energy is made, called cytochrome, which uses light to increase production of cellular energy. LLLT may act on this. Laser light also increases levels of anti-inflammatory immune chemicals and modulates the immune system by decreasing production of neutrophils, which attack potential threats, while increasing the "garbage collectors" known as macrophages.

The doctor this chapter discusses, Dr Khan, had treated a number of women with endometriosis, in some cases so well they could cancel surgery. A specialist in neuroplasticity discussed in the book's prequel, Barbara Arrowsmith Young, had her postsurgical adhesions from endometriosis surgery healed by LLLT. Previously, every operation would make her scarring worse and she developed chronic pain and monthly bowel obstructions. The LLLT treatment meant she was able to travel again too, as the bowel obstructions were often dangerous. Dr Khan had even controlled endometriosis in patients so well that some could cancel surgeries!

How far can LLLT go? One case discussed, "Gary", had been totally blind and deaf after inflammation from meningitis damaged his brain. After a few treatments, he began to regain touch sensations around his ears. After two months, he began to perceive light and sound for the first time in ten years. These were indistinct – shadows and silhouettes clicking in and out; the "outline" of a word – but were progress, and would take several years to become something substantial. Other patients had enjoyed significant relief from depression, enough to return to work and reduce their medication. This is from inflammation becoming "unblocked".

I could never forget the healing powers of therapies like LLLT and PEMF from when I first learnt of them, in my early days of writing for other natural health businesses. My first encounter was while writing an article on how to speed up fracture healing, inspired by the dismally slow recovery times of my classmates in high school. An animal study showed that LLLT significantly increased the number of osteoblasts (bone-building cells) and bone volume, as well as raising bending stiffness and maximum force by up to four times compared to the non-lasered group.

A review of clinical trials on PEMF and LIPUS (low-intensity pulsed ultrasound), another regenerative therapy, found significant effects in humans. One of the papers reviewed found a reduction in healing time of 12 days among non-smokers treated with LIPUS (84 days versus 96 days) for clinical healing, and a reduction of 33 days for healing with PEMF (96 days instead of 129). Even in smokers using these therapies, healing time was reduced to 103 days from 175 (the control group's time) using LIPUS, and to 96 days from 175 using PEMF. This is without other treatment, such as ensuring increased protein intake. I had to add this effect of therapies such as LLLT, PEMF and LIPUS in because while sports injuries are common, pain, disability and the side effects of drugs and surgery are just downright nasty.

Spending Time in Nature

It's almost instinctive that spending time in natural environments, whether they be land or water, can benefit our health. Beyond just feeling good and internet memes calling forests an antidepressant, however, is years of research and clinical experience. In fact, the term *shinrin-yoku*, or forest bathing, was coined in 1982 to describe making contact with and taking in the atmosphere of forests. Then, in 2007, the Japanese Society of Forest Medicine was established to promote the research and practice of spending time in nature as a therapeutic tool.

Infla-Menses

One of these studies is a series of field experiments from 2010, which involved a total of 280 healthy university-age men who took turns walking in and viewing both a forest and city environment. It turned out that spending time in the forest resulted in lower cortisol, blood pressure and pulse rate, as well as greater dominance of the parasympathetic nervous system over the sympathetic side. The sympathetic (SNS) and parasympathetic (PSNS) nervous systems are the two sides of the autonomic nervous system, which controls our automatic physical processes. The SNS is known as the "fight or flight" side, while the PSNS is referred to as the "rest and digest" part. Therefore, spending time in nature may improve digestion and tissue repair, as well as regulating immunity through reducing excess cortisol.

The men also showed improvements in their POMS scores, which measures mood. Tension-anxiety, depression, fear, anger-hostility and confusion scores all significantly fell, while vigour rose, when they were in the forests. Exposure to city environments worsened these scores. This means forest-bathing may help people with mental and emotional issues as part of a holistic treatment plan. In another study of men with heart issues, inflammation fell, protection against oxidative stress rose, and POMS scores improved in the forest-bathing men. The opposite effect was found in those visiting a city, with their oxidative stress spiking and POMS scores improving far less.

Direct contact with the earth, especially through natural bodies of water, also provides us with antioxidant support that can protect against the oxidative effects of pollutants. This method of "supplementation" is quite popular with my friends; one always thanks the earth when he swims in the sea or a lake. But why? Spending time in or near the water exposes us to negatively charged ions, so a walk on the beach can be the perfect mini digital detox. Whether salty or fresh, moving water breaks up air molecules. Russian researchers have found that negative ions can stimulate production of our antioxidant enzymes, including superoxide dismutase, which helps to break the oxidation-inflammation cycle. Additionally, a study by Columbia University found that negative ion exposure could in fact be as effective as antidepressants, so they may help beat the PMS blues. Negative ions boost oxygen supply to the brain, an essential resource for survival, healing and our mental energy.

Swimming, particularly if the water is cold, may be even better than activities on or near water – unless you have your period and getting cold causes cramps. In that case, it's best to wait until it's over. Compared to those who don't, people who swim in winter were found to have higher levels of their own antioxidants. Here's an interesting fact: declining levels of one, known as catalase, contributes to grey hair! Glutathione was 20% higher in winter swimmers, while less of it was temporarily used up (oxidised). This, however, was in Berlin, where they swam for around five minutes, and never more than ten. If you live in a colder region such as this, stay safe! If you live in a warmer climate, "cold" water can be safe for longer periods of time, and you are likely to still get at least some effect due to the temperature change. The definition of cold in this case was 1-5 degrees Celsius, while cold in a tropical or subtropical area – such as where I live – can mean 15-20 degrees.

Infla-Menses

The reason why cold water swimming works is that it "hardens" the body. Acting as a short-term, natural stressor, it stimulates production of our own antioxidants by temporarily increasing oxidative stress. This may either teach the body to keep antioxidant levels high in preparation for the future, or it's in our nature to over-compensate unless overloaded. A similar method has even been used with young children in Siberia, to help them stay strong and healthy over winter! Teachers noted far fewer infections with a daily routine of exercises, 90 seconds of outdoor water play, and time in a sauna.

If your inflammatory issues extend to atopic conditions affecting your respiratory system or skin, sea water may be helpful in another aspect. Centuries ago, people stopped fearing and started enjoying the ocean because doctors would recommend seaside holidays as treatment for various illnesses, including skin and respiratory problems. Patients developed a taste for it over time, and enjoying Vitamin Sea has become a normal part of life for an increasing number of people. Ocean water contains more minerals, such as sodium chloride (salt), magnesium and calcium, compared to most fresh water. Many people with eczema and psoriasis report improvements after ocean swimming, although it is irritating to others. This may depend on local magnesium content, pollution and individual sensitivities.

Sea water also has mild antiseptic properties. I always noticed clearer skin after acne breakouts, but don't swim without a dressing over wounds or broken skin. It's more of a preventive measure, and is much like the use of mildly antimicrobial foods to prevent overgrowth of harmful intestinal bacteria. Don't worry about sea water disrupting the healthy skin microbiome, either. Your skin was made to take some natural "punishment", and even in the less hardy intestinal lining, it takes months of consistently sticking to a new diet in order to really change the microbiome. As for respiratory health, sea water is a soothing anti-inflammatory, and Allergy UK's director of clinical services states that those living near and swimming in the sea have healthier respiratory systems. Exercise in natural environments has greater mental health benefits anyway.

Sleep Hygiene

Many of us read off of e-readers, play video games or watch TV right before bed, and worse still are those of us who do these things until the early hours of the morning! But when I had a client who complained of poor energy and couldn't afford her herbal prescription for another few weeks, one of my major recommendations was for her to stop using her phone 1-2 hours before bed. This was the biggest lifestyle change she made, and it quickly led to significant improvements in her energy and overall wellbeing.

So how does cutting back on the use of electronic devices improve sleep quality, and along with it, energy? The light emitting from these devices is higher in short wavelengths of light, meaning it has more "blue" light, and this has a greater effect on melatonin levels than any other wavelength. Melatonin is a hormone that aids sleep length and quality, which is why it is meant to be present at low levels during the day, begin its release a few hours before bed, and peak in the middle of the night. Light suppresses melatonin production, and humans are most sensitive to blue light.

Infla-Menses

A 2014 study compared the biological effects of reading a printed book versus an e-reader before bed, in order to see if these theories were correct. Volunteers who read e-books took longer to fall asleep, had lower melatonin levels and were less alert in the morning than people who read printed books. Being in the habit of using electronic devices before bed can also raise the risk of developing sleep-onset insomnia. On the other hand, the shorter time it took for people to fall asleep after reading print books was the same as a drug tested for patients with primary insomnia! To make things worse for night owls, melatonin is a natural antidepressant. Disrupting our circadian rhythms is detrimental to mood and brain plasticity.

Melatonin is also a powerful antioxidant, anti-inflammatory and immunomodulator. In fact, all immune cell types respond to it. This is why supporting its natural rhythms can be helpful in cases of endometriosis and PCOS. Laboratory studies have found that melatonin reduces COX-2, and can shrink endometriotic lesions in rats. As for human women with the disease, a phase II clinical trial demonstrated that it can be effective in relieving pelvic pain. Compared to the placebo it successfully reduced period pain, daily pain and pain during urination or bowel movements. Much of the development of PCOS is tied to oxidative stress, which damages the egg cells. Melatonin not only helps them mature (so they don't form cysts) by keeping inflammation and oxidation down, but also by regulating hormonal balance. What's more, it can protect the liver from the harmful effects of PCOS.

We still need more clinical studies on melatonin for endometriosis and PCOS, but with the benefits of keeping good sleep habits for our overall health, it's best not to disrupt our natural rhythms. If you can't avoid staying up late on a computer (such as if you are studying), you can download a blue light-blocker. I use the free app f.lux on my laptop.

Saunas and Sweating

Sauna "bathing" is a time-honoured tradition from many cultures around the world, taking different forms and purposes by region. If you've never experienced it before, their appeal may seem hard to understand, but they really do feel amazing when you've found the right type for you! I have been to an old Istanbul hammam, built in the 1590s, where the women's and men's sections consist mostly of a huge steam room with taps and basins on the sides. You splash the water over yourself using shallow bowls to get clean and cool off, and your attendant uses it too when she scrubs you and washes your hair. Afterwards, you shower before leaving. Bathhouses in less arid European countries often involve a sauna at the beginning, but you progress through several rooms to a very cold swim that finishes off the sequence.

So ... *why?* Besides the obvious, that the vast majority of people did not have their own baths or showers until the 20th century, the bathhouses we know today exist because use of a sauna or steam room has many health benefits. A study on Finnish men found that regular sauna bathing, between four and seven sessions per week, significantly reduced inflammatory markers and excessive white blood cell populations. These effects held at the 11-year follow up, as they most likely maintained their habits.

One of the mechanisms behind the benefits of sweating is enhanced detoxification. For example, phthalates have been found in sweat but often not in urine or blood, meaning they aren't efficiently removed from the body by other means. These are in soft plastics as well as conventional cosmetics. The infamous BPA can be removed by sweating too, even in people who can't detoxify it through other routes. Yet another group of persistent toxins that sweating removes is the flame retardant PDBEs. Different flame retardants are best excreted through different ways of working up a sweat. PBDE 28 is removed the most by exercise, PBDE 100 is best removed by infrared sauna, and steam sauna is best for PBDE 153. As for heavy metals, cadmium, lead, arsenic and mercury are safely excreted by sweating.

Whether you choose a sauna, steam room or exercise, sweating can be effective, but use it responsibly – don't spend more time in saunas or steam rooms than recommended and stay hydrated. It's best to wash or dry the sweat off too, to prevent reabsorption.

Self-Mastery

Have you ever had something go wrong in your life, or be affected by setbacks, and have a well-meaning friend or relative tell you that it isn't "meant to be"? Have you ever been pressured to believe in something like fate or biological determinism (especially if you, like me, are childfree and pro-peace)? We are often told that it is "comforting" to think in these ways, but in fact, the opposite is true. It turns out that need to have power over our lives to achieve optimal health in every way: physical, mental, emotional and spiritual.

The most popular psychological model of behavior that I studied in my degree was Self-Determination Theory (SDT). All human beings have three basic psychological needs: autonomy, competency, and relatedness. Autonomy means being the master of your life and destiny, and is a universal need across all cultures. SDT also differentiates between intrinsic and extrinsic motivation: motivation by internal drives (e.g. personal values) versus motivation by rewards (e.g. money or approval). You can be autonomously motivated by both intrinsic and extrinsic factors, if the extrinsic rewards are aligned with your sense of self. For example, I value my independence and therefore want to earn my own money, and would prefer to be well-known rather than obscure in order to help others. The opposite of autonomy, on the psychological level, is learned helplessness.

Learned helplessness is the state of feeling like you have little to no control over your life. Many people with chronic illnesses feel this way, as statements like "incurable", "irreversible" and so on are constantly drilled into their heads, but could this be a self-fulfilling prophecy? In a study of people with rheumatoid arthritis, those with a high degree of learned helplessness had significantly worse scores as measured by the Health Assessment Questionnaire (HAQ), compared to average volunteers. Patients with a low degree of learned helplessness had significantly better scores. Median HAQ scores were 0.25 in the low helplessness group, 0.88 in the "normal" group, and 1.63 in the high learned

Infla-Menses

helplessness group. Rheumatoid arthritis is an autoimmune condition where a dysregulated immune system attacks the joints, resulting in the pain and swelling of chronic inflammation, as well as often severe disability. Yet another reason to pay attention to what your menstrual cycle is telling you now, instead of waiting for it to worsen and spill over into other aspects of your health.

Self-mastery so often requires us to recognise and heal all parts of ourselves. We may need to consider an entirely different perspective on what makes us human. Healer Kageni Njeru explains that "In the shamanistic point of view, we are more than just a physical being; we have a soul within". "When we work as healers and shamans, we work from a place where we know there is a physical body; a mental body where thoughts, beliefs and programming are kept; the emotional body and the spirit body. This can be expanded more into other ethereal bodies."

Kageni adds that there is much we have forgotten about the physical body: "There is a flow of energy (prana, chi, etc.), the purest form of love from the Divine. It is a constant stream, but topped up every morning. Once it comes through your crown, the body is to receive love and emit to the world." She explains that this light must be distributed by a complex network of energetic systems, such as the meridian lines or chakras. "You are the breaker switch; you transform it into a kind of creation to share with the world (books, art, teaching etc.). The Soul essence is different, and is projected as you create it."

We are truly powerful beings. When I started to perform energy healing, I noticed a shift in my own perspective even

180

while I was only practicing with free sessions for friends. I stopped seeing those who need healing as passive patients who should be babied. Instead, I started seeing "patients" as powerful individuals who deserve wholeness and just need support to get there.

But why spirituality? Psychological theories that only consider the material can leave us feeling more powerless and confused if we don't fit into their explanations. Looking at evolutionary psychology, we are told that pressures to reproduce and survive at least long enough to do so are what shape our brains. At worst, it can justify strict gender roles, racism and other power hierarchies, or you may just feel like you don't belong if you don't want children, thrive with diversity or you're a free spirit.

As we are all of Creation, burying who you are in response to the belief that conformity and obedience are necessary to get along with others does nothing to advance our consciousness-based evolution. Diversity is in fact our strength, and you can never be replaced nor replicated. Reclaim your inner power, and you will attract those you resonate with, who may be more diverse than you expected – I have friends from around the world, ranging in age from their early 20s to 70s. From experience I also notice that I am no longer as bothered by people I don't gel with, as long as they aren't forcing their will onto others.

If you have trouble conceptualising our non-material aspects, Kageni explains it as, "When you walk in the sun and see the rays, but don't feel the UV until it burns you, it is like the part of the body invisible to human eye. That's why you pick people's vibes. Look at it like a modem (physical), then you have this Wi-Fi around you (spirit body)."

Part of embracing our spiritual side is learning how to listen to our intuition. Doing so is very empowering, as you learn to make decisions without manipulation or other outside influence, and can more effectively evaluate advice from others. That is how I started to write this book; there was an inner knowing that I had to do it. Kageni explains this as "Not listening with your ears – it is intuiting, sensing, knowing and using all senses. Some would say 'listen with your eyes, listen with your feelings'... When you listen with your entire being, something will tell you, 'This person is lying to you', for example. Your inner being is feeling a disconnect of some kind."

She adds, "You have your innate, your consciousness and Higher Self. This part oversees all and knows what you're doing, knows where you're heading. You can never lie to it. All communicate to you through intuition. Your body is always talking to you, but are you listening? When you think, 'Something is missing; I've been feeling tired', it is often the first message something is wrong. We must start developing observation skills...You listen with your greater self, and to listen to your greater self." How many of us know someone who somehow *knew* they needed a second opinion from a doctor, or experienced it ourselves? How many of us have suffered medical emergencies after months or years of living *outside* of our self-mastery, and instead under other peoples' obligations?

Always remember what Kageni has to say about us as humans: "You are an individualised piece of God [Creation], a unique expression, different drops but form the ocean, we are one. This expression of you has never existed and will never exist again."

Starter Recipes for an Anti-Inflammatory Diet

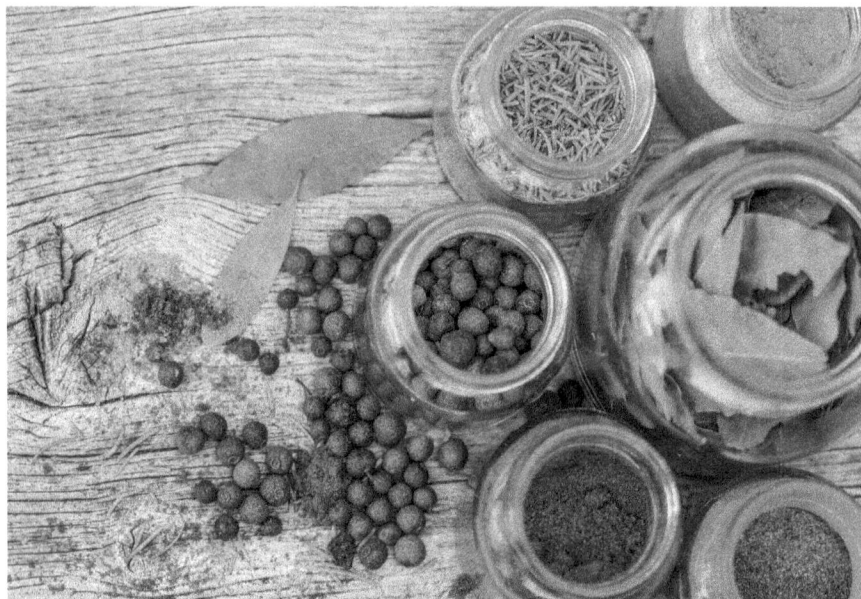

In English-speaking nations, we typically grew up with many inflammatory foods. Meat, white bread, flour-based cakes and snacks such as chips (crisps) have been the norm, but now we have access to a wide variety of healthier foods from other cultures and new ideas. Here are some ideas to get started, which you can make as a single serving or more if you're into meal prepping.

Cashew Yoghurt Breakfast Parfait

A cashew "yoghurt" parfait is an anti-inflammatory breakfast recipe rich in protein and healthy fats. To make the cashew yoghurt, you need:

- Two cups of cashews, which will give you two servings. Otherwise, just use ¾ or 1 cup.
- Juice from ¼ lemon (or ½ if small)
- 1 teaspoon of honey
- 1 teaspoon of natural thickener, such as psyllium husk

First, soak the cashews overnight. In the morning, add the lemon juice, honey and psyllium husks or other thickener to the portion you want to use, and refrigerate the rest. Blend, adding water if it gets too thick. Once it's smooth, spoon it into a bowl and add any healthy toppings, such as berries, hemp seeds and/or coconut flakes. You can try to copy the image kicking off the *Natural Remedies* section, for example. If you're craving chocolate or want extra flavour, you can add cacao powder to the yoghurt or its topping. In my case, Australian summers can call for the addition of mango!

Infla-Menses
Protein Powder Pancakes

Need protein, but don't want a heavy meal during your period? This recipe comes from a 2017 issue of *Connect Magazine*, a new-age publication in my local area. Combine:

- Half a mashed banana
- ¼ cup protein powder. I recommend a vegan, sprouted blend; it doesn't feel so heavy, but you can use whey if you tolerate it well. Whey is high in cysteine, an amino acid your body needs to make glutathione.
- 2 eggs, beaten (or a vegan substitute)
- 1 teaspoon of flaxseed (ground)
- Cinnamon or ginger, to taste.

Cook as you would any other pancake, and add fruit of your choice to taste. Top it with more fruit, yoghurt or a dairy-free alternative.

Vegan Cashew Cream Cheese

This recipe comes from my friend Ebony Mombaerts, and is one that she developed for her vegan food business, Intrusting Delights. You can use it as a substitute for dairy cheese in any meal that would typically call for it, or just as a snack with chips. The ingredients are:

- Two handfuls of raw cashews
- Two cloves of garlic
- A decent pinch of salt
- Water to just cover the cashews

Just blend it all together and serve! You can also add nutritional yeast, or sesame seeds for extra calcium.

Infla-Menses
Simple Cauliflower Soup

This is another recipe from Ebony, which you can use as an entrée (starter) or side dish. To make up to eight servings, depending on how much you want, you need:

- One large cauliflower
- Two cups of coconut cream
- Coconut oil
- 1 teaspoon of cumin
- 1 teaspoon of turmeric
- 1 teaspoon paprika
- Salt and pepper to taste

Chop the cauliflower and cook it in coconut oil, then add a pinch of salt and coconut cream. Continue cooking until the cauliflower is soft. Take it off the stove and blend it with a hand blender, adding the spices and pepper.

Cauliflower Curry

This is a North Indian-style dish based on another seen in *The Higher Taste.* Here, I replaced potatoes with chickpeas and added pepitas for extra protein and zinc. It can be served with rice, salad, or a gluten-free flatbread or toast. For roughly four servings, you need:

- One medium-sized cauliflower, cut into small florets
- One can of diced tomatoes, or two blanched and diced fresh ones.
- 400 grams of cooked chickpeas (canned or done yourself)
- One handful of green pepitas
- ½ teaspoon black mustard seeds
- 1 teaspoon cumin seeds
- Two chillies, seeded and diced
- 1 teaspoon ginger, fresh or powdered
- ½ teaspoon turmeric
- ½ teaspoon garam masala (check for gluten)
- 2 teaspoons dried coriander
- 2 tablespoons fresh parsley or more coriander

Heat oil in a large saucepan, and first add the mustard seeds. When these start to pop (be careful, they can jump high!), add the cumin seeds and saute them until they darken. Add the chillies and ginger, and saute them for a few moments again before adding in the cauliflower and chickpeas. Cook for 4-5 minutes, mixing the ingredients together. Stir in the tomatoes, turmeric, garam masala, dried coriander and pepitas. Cover and simmer for 10-15 minutes, stirring occasionally, and add more water if necessary. Sprinkle with the fresh parsley or coriander to serve.

Infla-Menses
Channa Masala

This is an easy version of Channa Masala adapted from a recipe on the BBC website, and like the cauliflower curry above, it is helpful for when you need to pre-plan meals. Here, for three or four servings, you need:

- 400g can of chickpeas, or the pre-soaked equivalent
- One onion, finely chopped
- 400g of canned or roughly diced tomatoes
- One clove of garlic
- 2-2.5cm fresh ginger, or dried equivalent
- One roughly chopped chilli
- 1tbsp of coconut oil
- ¾ cup of plant milk; here I used organic rice milk
- 1tsp turmeric
- 1tsp garam masala (check label for added wheat)
- ½ tsp ground cumin
- ½ tsp ground coriander
- ½ tsp chilli powder
- Fresh coriander leaves to serve

First, either blitz the onions with garlic, ginger and chilli, or fry them in a large pan with the coconut oil. Stir in the other spices and cook for another minute once the onions have softened. Add the tomatoes and stir for another 2-5 minutes, depending on whether you are using fresh or canned tomatoes. Finally, add the chickpeas and plant milk, then cook for 10 more minutes. Serve with rice and sprinkled with fresh coriander; you can also use dairy or coconut yoghurt as another topping.

Chilli con Lentil Burrito Bowl

How to show your family that vegetarian dishes can be just as delicious as meat, or even better? I have you covered. This is a plant-based version of chilli *con carne* which replaces mince with red lentils, no processed meat substitutes required. For four or more servings:

- One cup of red lentils
- 400g of pre-soaked kidney beans
- 400g of diced tomatoes, canned or fresh
- 2 tablespoons passata
- One medium brown onion
- One fresh chilli, remove the seeds
- 1 ½ tablespoons paprika
- One crushed garlic clove or dried equivalent
- 1 heaped teaspoon each of cumin seeds
- 1 heaped teaspoon of coriander

- Optional base: a large handful of lettuce per serve and/or one cup of rice
- Optional garnishes: cheese, any sort of dairy or vegan; avocado and sour cream

First, boil the lentils until tender. Chop the onions, chilli and tomatoes (if fresh) while the lentils are cooking. When these are done, heat olive or coconut oil in a large saucepan and start cooking the onions, combining with the chilli, paprika, cumin and garlic after two minutes. Add lentils, kidney beans, tomatoes, passata and coriander; simmer after five minutes. Start cooking the rice and/or preparing the other ingredients, turn the saucepan off once heated through and serve!

Infla-Menses
Falafel Balls

Seen in kebab shops everywhere, falafel is a satisfying, protein-rich food mostly made of chickpeas. This recipe is based on that in *The Higher Taste*, where it is called "Israeli Chickpea Croquettes (Falafel)", but I added pepitas and buckwheat flour for extra nutrients. Pepitas, or shelled pumpkin seeds, are rich in zinc, a mineral commonly low in vegan and vegetarian diets. Buckwheat is high in protein and contains magnesium, iron and zinc. You need:

- 1 ¼ cups of raw chickpeas, soaked overnight and drained; or 1 400g can of chickpeas, drained.
- 2 ½ tablespoons of green pepitas
- 1 heaped tablespoon of buckwheat flour
- ½-1 teaspoon of garlic granules
- ¾ cup finely chopped parsley, or a liberal amount of dried parsley
- 1 teaspoon ground coriander or cardamom. The original recipe calls for coriander, but I didn't have any the first time I made this, so I used cardamom.
- 1 teaspoon ground cumin
- ¼ teaspoon cayenne pepper
- ½ teaspoon baking powder
- Salt and pepper to taste
- Sesame seeds

Mince the chickpeas and pepitas in a food processor. Scrape into a bowl, and add the buckwheat flour, spices, herbs, salt and baking powder. Mix these together and let it stand for 30 minutes. Form the mixture into 12 falafel balls, or up to 16 if you prefer them smaller. Coat them in sesame seeds. Finally, either heat olive oil in a pan and lightly fry them, or bake in an oven at 200 degrees C for 15-20 minutes. Serve with hummus and salad, rice with vegetables or as a gluten-free salad sandwich or wrap.

Infla-Menses
Injera

As I wrote above, injera is a traditional Ethiopian bread usually made with teff flour, an easy way to get enough protein, iron, zinc and calcium as a vegan or vegetarian. The ingredients are simply teff flour, water and salt, but recommended ratios vary.

SBS Food advises us to use 3 ½ cups of water for every ¾ cups of teff, while *Yum Universe* recommends 1 ½ cups of teff flour with 2 cups of water. Unless you know someone who makes injera themselves, you may have to experiment to find the ideal ratio for the flour available to you.

First, mix the teff flour with water and leave it standing for a day or two until it starts to bubble. Once ready, it is described by *SBS Food* as slightly sour with a crepe batter-like consistency. Add salt, and spoon portions of the mixture into a pre-heated pan, cooking it slowly. If you used a shorter fermentation time, add ½ a teaspoon of baking powder with the salt. Injera should be bubbly (like the Swiss cheese of breads) and not browned or too thick.

Vegan Keto Pizza Bases

One of the most loved foods, and one of the most missed when transitioning to a keto, vegan or otherwise anti-inflammatory diet, is pizza! Commercial gluten-free bases can be crumbly and full of highly refined grains, while many keto recipes are excessively rich and not suitable for those of us who can't have dairy foods. This simple recipe, from Carine of *Sweet as Honey*, solves all of these problems. For each base, you need:

- ¾ cup coconut flour
- 2 tablespoons ground psyllium husk
- 1 cup lukewarm water
- 1 tablespoon extra-virgin olive oil
- Salt, to taste.

First, preheat the oven to 220 degrees Celsius. Mix all ingredients together and then knead them with your hand for one minute. When it starts to dry out, roll all the dough into a ball and set it aside for ten minutes so the flours can continue to absorb the water.

The dough should be elastic enough now to be rolled. To prevent it from sticking to the rolling pin, place it between two oiled sheets of baking paper. Roll the dough until it reaches the thickness you want – a thin crust is a crispy crust, just like wheat bases! Take the top layer of baking paper off, and bake the base for 12-15 minutes as is, or use a cutter to make two or three mini bases. All random shapes are welcome here!

Infla-Menses

Finally, use whatever toppings you like, as long as they're compatible with your dietary needs. The original recipe suggests a tomato sauce made for pizzas, baby spinach, olives and mozzarella. As a kid, I remember going to a pizza shop with some of the most *interesting* toppings you could think of. If you think pineapple is strange, consider mango or crabmeat! Fresh pineapple is quite anti-inflammatory, so I'm all for it, but I don't judge regardless. Just heat it under the oven to melt the cheese, whether it be dairy or vegan.

Gluten Free Wraps

This recipe for gluten-free wraps is here thanks to Ebony, as we both sought something more awesome and nutritious than crumbly, refined commercial wraps. Here, you need:

- ½ cup of buckwheat flour
- ½ cup of tapioca flour
- ½ cup of besan (chickpea) flour
- ½ cup of brown rice flour
- 2 ½ cups of water
- Coconut oil for cooking

First, mix all the ingredients together. If it's too thick, add a tablespoon of water. Heat coconut oil in a large pan, about half a teaspoon of oil per wrap. Pour ¾ cup of the wrap mixture into the pan, then pick it up and move around to evenly spread the mix. Flip after one side has cooked well, and once they're done serve with whatever fillings you want.

Infla-Menses
Red Lentil Dahl

I find dried lentils to be a very cheap and versatile source of protein and iron, with a one kilogram bag yielding me over 10 servings. On top of this, Indian cuisine has gifted the world with some very anti-inflammatory recipes, which also taste great! This recipe serves four, perfect for meal prepping. You need:

- 1 ½ cups of dried red lentils
- 1 chopped onion
- 400g of diced tomatoes (average can size)
- 1 tablespoon each of turmeric and cumin seeds
- 1 or 2 tablespoons of ground ginger
- 1 teaspoon each of chilli (flakes or powder) and mustard seeds
- 3 or 4 minced garlic cloves, or dried equivalent
- A handful of baby spinach leaves

In a large pan, heat oil (such as coconut or high-quality olive oil), then add the onion and spices. When the onions have softened, add in the lentils and three metric cups of water. Once the lentils are almost fully cooked, add the tomatoes, and continue until the lentils are done. Turn the heat down so it is now simmering. Stir in the spinach leaves and allow them to wilt.

In a separate, small pot, start to boil one cup of rice after you've added the lentils to the other saucepan. Turn off once the rice is thoroughly cooked; you can taste test it with a couple of grains. When everything is finished, you can serve the dahl with plain yoghurt (dairy or vegan) and/or mango chutney.

Spinach and Flax Keto Crumpets

This recipe is adapted from The Charlie Foundation, an organisation dedicated to ketogenic diet therapies. For this easy breakfast or lunch, you need:

- One large egg, whisked
- 22 grams of oil (e.g. olive, liquid coconut oil, hemp seed)
- 13 grams flaxseed meal
- 11 grams of finely chopped, raw baby spinach
- 1 teaspoon of baking powder
- Keto-permitted toppings of your choice. The original recipe calls for butter; I prefer basil pesto, avocado and sardines.

First, weigh the oil, flaxseed meal and spinach to ensure accuracy, and mix all ingredients except for the toppings in a bowl. Then, line a baking dish with paper and pour in the mixture. Cook at 180 degrees Celsius (fan-forced) for 15-20 minutes, or until it just starts to turn golden brown. Add toppings and enjoy with herbal tea.

Infla-Menses
Split Pea Vege Burgers

If you want a burger but (like me) aren't a fan of the processed commercial varieties, make your own! Split peas are high in protein, and like all grains or legumes I recommend you purchase organically-grown ones. For four to six burger patties, you need:

- One cup of dried split peas
- One medium brown onion, finely chopped
- ¼ cup buckwheat flour if it is too moist
- 2 eggs or vegan equivalent
- Your preferred blend of herbs and spices. Here, I used sumac, oregano, thyme and sesame seeds, similar to the *za'atar* blend.
- A sprinkle of coconut flour if the mixture is too moist

Boil the split peas until cooked, then rinse and drain. Then, combine all ingredients in a food processor and pulse. Form the mixture into patties and refrigerate for 10 minutes so they can set. Finally, fry them in a small amount of olive or coconut oil until browned (but not blackened). It's up to you which type of bread, if any, you use, and what salad vegetables go with it. I like to have these with lettuce, tomato, mushrooms, tomato sauce and dijon mustard, of course on gluten-free bread.

Steamed Fish

Steaming is one of the healthiest ways to cook fish, as it cuts down on AGE formation. This is quite common in Southeast Asian cuisine, so you will find many flavour combinations far more interesting than crumbing and frying your fish. As a general guide:

First, invest in a bamboo steaming basket, and line it with baking paper. Aluminium foil is may leach into food, which may come back to bite us later.

Then, choose your fish! The Australian Heart Foundation lists fish by EPA+DHA content, with winners including bream, rainbow trout and salmon (Atlantic and Australian). As for avoiding excessive mercury, the Natural Resources Defence Council cautions against shark, mackerel, swordfish and other very large species. Coal burning, and to a lesser extent natural trace amounts, are responsible for its accumulation.

As for marinade, you can play it simple with lemon juice and zest, or use a combination of herbs and spices. These can include chilli, tamarind, ginger, turmeric, galangal (related to ginger and turmeric), coriander, dill or fennel. You can also crush nuts and sprinkle them on top of the fish, such as peanuts or pistachios.

Alternatives to chips or mashed potatoes and peas include sweet potato chips; stir-fried vegetables, such as bok choy, capsicum (bell pepper), onions and carrots; or zucchini noodles and pesto. On hot days, however, a salad can be the best.

Infla-Menses
Stuffed Mushrooms

This recipe is my mother's invention, from when she wanted to cook for my birthday party but had to cater for my vegan friends. These, along with the two other vegan dishes, were even loved by the meat-eating guests, so I had to write the recipe down for future use. Amounts are meant to be taken as a guide, as when I asked she had forgotten exactly how much of each ingredient she used.

- 6 portobello mushrooms
- 2-3 finely chopped zucchini, depending on size
- Tomato paste, enough to coat the zucchini
- Several shallots, chopped
- Flat leaf parsley, chopped, ¼ cup or to taste
- 1 teaspoon each of sugar, allspice and garlic
- Salt and pepper

It's quite easy, really. Stir-fry all ingredients, and then stuff them into the portobello mushrooms and bake for 20-30 minutes at 200 degrees C.

Vegan Nachos

Vegan nachos are an easy way in which to use nutritional yeast, as well as ensure an adequate protein intake. You can make more or less of them for one, two or even three servings, so you don't have to cook before every meal. To prepare nachos healthier than how you may have learnt in middle school:

- Start with a base of quality corn chips. Brands vary by country, but aim for those with a simple, natural ingredient list, preferably with organic corn.
- Spoon a liberal amount of tomato salsa on top. Use the same above guidelines for buying pre-prepared salsa, or this recipe. Add chilli to taste.
- Add around 400g of kidney beans (typical can size). Soak them first if you bought them dried!
- Finally, top it with vegan cheese. One recipe from *Minimalist Baker* combines ¾ cups of cashews with three tablespoons of nutritional yeast. You can add garlic and salt like this recipe, or mustard like some others use. Of course, you can increase the amounts of these ingredients depending on your needs, but stick to the ratio. When you're done, heat under an oven and enjoy with salad.

Infla-Menses
Mediterranean Zu-ccine

Ebony's Mediterranean zu-ccine is a perfect low-carb substitute for conventional wheat or gluten-free pasta. For three or four servings, you need:

- Three or four zucchinis
- ½ yellow and ½ red large capsicum (bell pepper)
- Five asparagus stalks
- ½ red onion
- One can of champignons
- 400g can of diced tomato
- 1 teaspoon of curry powder
- 1 teaspoon of sage
- 3-4 tablespoons of coconut oil

First, use a vegetable peeler to fettuccine the zucchini; make them even by peeling each side of the zucchini. Mildly salt your pasta over a strainer. Cut up and fry the end and last thin pieces.

Then, cut the asparagus up into 5 pieces, putting the heads aside, and dice the onion. Put onion, asparagus and little bits of zucchini to fry on high with a tablespoon of oil. Cut up capsicum into cubes and champignons in half each; add this and the asparagus heads once the above is cooked well. After about five minutes, add the zucchini and turn the heat right down, toss softly and put the lid on for a few minutes. Add tomato, and simmer with the lid on for a few more minutes. Serve with vegan cashew cream cheese or yeast flakes, and with whatever protein source you want.

Golden Milk

We now know that turmeric can be a powerful anti-inflammatory, but if you don't want to take pills or capsules, and prefer to use food as medicine, I recommend golden milk as a home remedy. There are a few variations, but typically involves the following; similar to Dr Weil's recipe:

- 2 cups of milk. Can be cow, goat, hemp, coconut etc. as long as it has some fat content.
- 1 tablespoon of powdered or fresh peeled, grated turmeric.
- Black pepper, usually around three or four peppercorns.
- ½ tablespoon fresh grated ginger (powder can suffice here too if necessary).
- Optional: ¼ - 1 teaspoon of cinnamon, add to taste.

To make golden milk, mix and heat the ingredients; stir well; and simmer for ten minutes. Then, strain it and, if you want, add honey to sweeten it. Remember to use organic ingredients where possible, and the strong flavours may make it an acquired taste.

Infla-Menses
Healthy Homemade Mocha

Many women prefer warm drinks during their period, which is also seen as the perfect occasion to indulge in chocolate. (how many of us who don't even get cravings have used that as an excuse?) However, we want to avoid processed drinks and ingredients that are full of added sugar and chemical additives, so here is one alternative:

- Boiled water
- 1 teaspoon of coffee, or dandelion root-based substitute
- 1 teaspoon raw cacao powder
- ½ - 1 teaspoon high-quality honey (I use Manuka honey, at a lower food-grade strength)
- Splash of your preferred milk, whether it be organic dairy or plant-based.

Simply boil the water, add all ingredients and stir.

Kefir

Kefir is a tart, slightly fizzy fermented milk drink that originated in the Caucasus, a mountainous region that divides Europe and Asia. It's traditionally made from cow's milk, but you can find or make it from goat, sheep or even coconut milk! While fermented foods like kefir are credited for the relatively high populations of centenarians in the Caucasus, and while some over 110 – or even over 120, according to a practitioner specialising in parasite cleanses I met once! – may have the national ID to show for it, they aren't for everyone. Please consult a healthcare professional if you are immunocompromised (just as you would for probiotics), have a digestive disorder such as IBS, or are lactose intolerant.

If you want to make it, you need "kefir grains", which are tiny, rubbery structures made of the bacterial and yeast species that turn milk into kefir. They're like the scoby you use for kombucha. One you've sourced these, add a teaspoon of the grains to a glass of milk, cover it, and let it sit for 24 hours at room temperature. Kefir does best with full fat milk. Even though you can make it with low fat milk, the grains may lose their strength over time; it's the same thing with plant milks.

For safety and best results (according to The Kitchn), keep their fermentation temperature between 15 and 32 degrees Celsius (60 and 90 degrees Fahrenheit), and only use glass jars (metal spoons and strainers are fine). Any hotter than 32 degrees C/90 degrees F, and the milk will spoil. Afterwards, just strain out the grains so you can reuse them or store them by refrigerating them in a glass of milk.

Infla-Menses

The kefir should be about as thick as buttermilk, and tangy like yoghurt.

Another safety disclaimer: if you don't feel confident making it or keeping it within the safe temperature range isn't realistic, it's best to buy kefir. If you do want to make your own, get someone with experience to help you at first. Whether you made or bought it, you can enjoy kefir straight up; in smoothies; in lassis, a sweet Indian yoghurt drink with fruit or rosewater; or like doogh, with cucumber, mint, salt and ice.

Blueberry Spirulina Smoothie

This smoothie is inspired by a stem cell-enhancing supplement that has shown beneficial effects on inflammation and production of new neurons in pre-clinical research. One day after a tough workout, I decided to experiment on myself and make this better-than-coffee energy booster. You need:

- One banana
- A handful of blueberries
- 1 teaspoon of matcha powder
- ¼ - ½ teaspoon of spirulina powder, ensure this is organic and from a clean source
- Almond or hemp milk
- Manuka honey, to taste
- Optional: protein powder, one tablespoon or up to one recommended serving.

Cut the banana into small pieces and add combine it in your mixer with the blueberries, honey, spirulina, matcha and protein powder, if you're using it. Pour the almond or hemp milk over until these ingredients are covered. Then, blend all ingredients together until you have a smoothie! If you're planning on uploading a photo to Instagram, aim to find blue spirulina powder for the look, as its brilliant hue blends well with blueberries. Regular bright green spirulina is perfectly fine. Enjoy in the sun for a vitamin D boost, unless of course it's raining or you've already spent enough time out.

Infla-Menses
Mango Pineapple Smoothie

Perfect for summer, I adapted this one from a recipe on *Food Matters* a few years ago. Anti-inflammatory ginger, cinnamon and pineapple working together mean that you don't have to miss out on a fun beach day. For one larger serving or two smaller ones, you need:

- One cup of frozen mango (cubed)
- ½ cup of pineapple; it can be fresh or frozen but be sure to keep the core.
- 100mL of coconut milk
- ½ teaspoon ground ginger
- ½ teaspoon ground cinnamon
- Coconut flakes or hemp seeds to garnish.

Just combine all of the ingredients in a blender, garnish and enjoy! It is best to keep this smoothie away from meals if you want to maximise the anti-inflammatory benefits, because the bromelain in pineapple cores will contribute to protein digestion instead of relieving systemic inflammation. Of course, if you'd prefer a digestive aid, then don't separate it from meals.

Think Pink Smoothie

How was I going to use the rest of a pomegranate? This sweet and tart smoothie contains strawberries and pomegranate, two red fruits each with their own benefits. Strawberries are the top source of fistein, and pomegranates have a precursor to urolithin A, two substances that can boost cellular health and may help prevent consequences of damage such as inflammation. The ingredients are just:

- One medium banana
- About ¼ of a pomegranate's seeds
- 2-4 strawberries, depending on size
- Plant milk, such as almond or hemp

Cut the banana and strawberries into small slices, and combine with the pomegranate seeds into your mixer of choice. Pour plant milk in until they are just covered, and blend together until smooth. Dress it up with another strawberry, because a lemon wedge is a little cliched and out of place here.

Appendix: Diet Diary and Cycle Chart

To help you take charge of your health, I have included a daily diet diary and cycle chart. You can photocopy as many of each as you need, and ask to enlarge them if they are too small. If you want full-colour versions, contact me through my website (the address is in the copyright page).

The purpose of each is to provide an easy to read measurement of your baseline state of health, and what improvements you make with dietary, lifestyle and other natural interventions. This helps you and your holistic health professional of choice to see what works best for you as an individual.

DAILY DIET DIARY

TODAY IS: DAY OF CYCLE:

BREAKFAST

LUNCH

DINNER

Infla-Menses

DAILY DIET DIARY

TODAY IS: DAY OF CYCLE:

DRINKS AND SNACKS

PHYSICAL ACTIVITY

GENERAL HEALTH NOTES

CYCLE CHART

KEY:
P = PERIOD   LF = LIGHT FLOW   MF = MODERATE FLOW
HF = HEAVY FLOW   SP = SPOTTING   CL = CLOTTING   FL =
FLOODING   DD = DUE DATE   DYS = PAIN   BA = BACKACHE
EM = EMOTIONALITY   A = ANXIETY   D = DEPRESSION   WR =
WATER RETENTION   CR = SUGAR CRAVINGS   APP = INCREASED
APPETITE   F = FATIGUE   HA = HEADACHE   M = MIGRAINE   CO
= COGNITIVE ISSUES   IN = INSOMNIA

DAYS

1	2	3
4	5	6
7	8	9

Infla-Menses

10	11	12
13	14	15
16	17	18
19	20	21
22	23	24

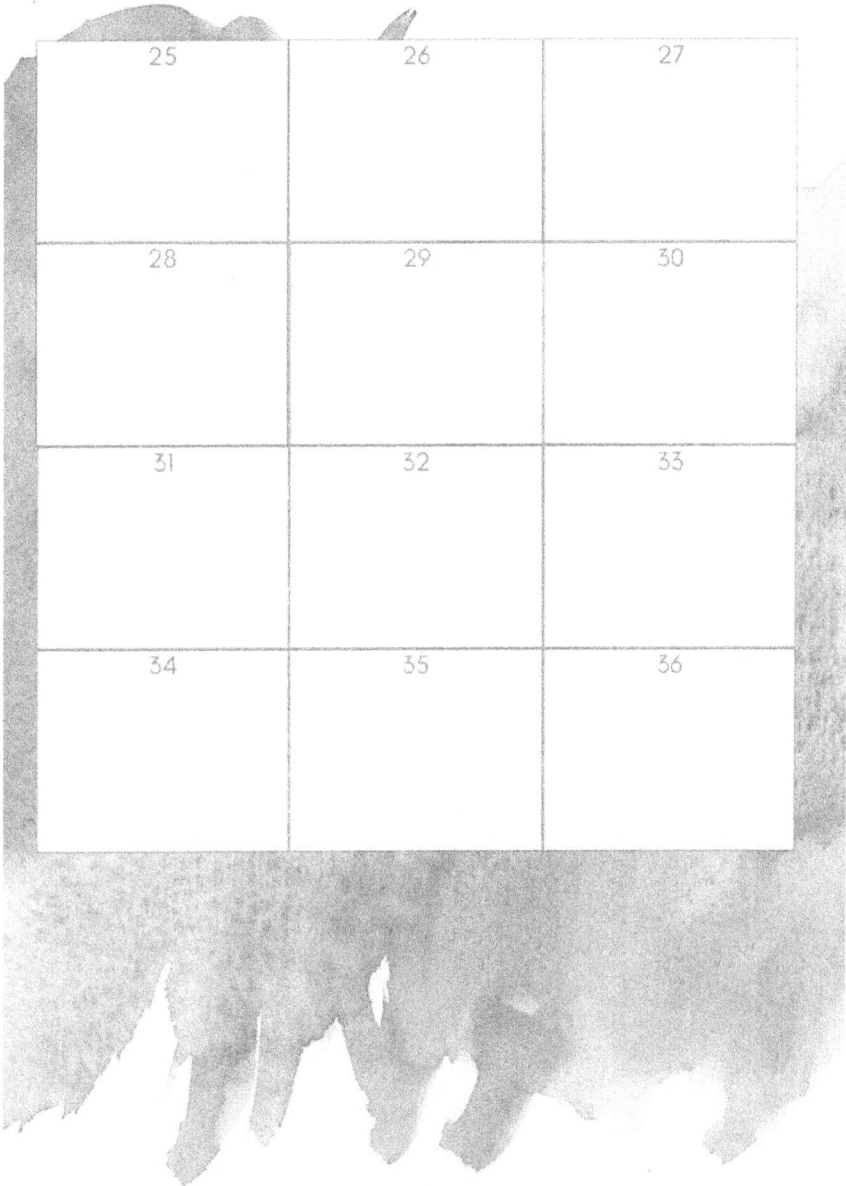

25	26	27
28	29	30
31	32	33
34	35	36

Infla-Menses

References

The Menstrual Cycle and Inflammation

Hechtman, L. (2014). *Clinical Naturopathic Medicine*. Elsevier.

https://www.sciencedirect.com/book/9780323035064/pediatric-clinical-advisor

https://www.tandfonline.com/doi/abs/10.3109/09513599509160464

https://www.liebertpub.com/doi/10.1089/jwh.2015.5529

https://www.ncbi.nlm.nih.gov/pmc/articles/PMC4890701/

https://www.ncbi.nlm.nih.gov/pmc/articles/PMC5791154/

Bredesen, D. (2017). *The End of Alzheimer's*. Vermilion.

https://www.ncbi.nlm.nih.gov/pmc/articles/PMC2077876/

http://doi.org/10.1186/s13075-015-0784-1

http://doi.org/10.1155/2018/4128984

https://link.springer.com/article/10.1007%2Fs10616-010-9326-5

Trickey, R. (2011). *Women, hormones and the menstrual cycle*. Third edition. Trickey Enterprises.

Bone, K., Carroll, L., Steels, E., & Newton, T. (2019, 6th April). *Metabolic Dysfunction: New Insights into Pathology Markers and Clinical Treatment of a Multifaceted Epidemic*. Seminar presented by Mediherb at the Sofitel Gold Coast Broadbeach, Queensland.

https://www.ncbi.nlm.nih.gov/pubmed/30538082/

https://www.ncbi.nlm.nih.gov/pmc/articles/PMC3245829/

https://www.hindawi.com/journals/mi/2018/9076485/

https://www.sciencedirect.com/science/article/abs/pii/S1465324917305261

Infla-Menses

https://ncbi.nlm.nih.gov/pmc/articles/PMC4152895/

What Causes Inflammation?

The Modern Western Diet:

https://www.ncbi.nlm.nih.gov/pmc/articles/PMC2868080/

https://www.clinicalnutritionjournal.com/article/S0261-5614(18)32540-8/fulltext

https://www.cell.com/cell/fulltext/S0092-8674%2817%2931493-9

https://www.nature.com/articles/srep00196

Red Meat:

http://www.onegreenplanet.org/animalsandnature/beef-eaters-plant-eaters-land-resources/

https://www.sciencedirect.com/book/9780323046015/mosbys-guide-to-womens-health

https://www.ajog.org/article/S0002-9378(18)30444-7/fulltext

https://epi.grants.cancer.gov/diet/foodsources/fatty_acids/table4.html

http://doi.org/10.1093/humrep/deq044

https://doi.org/10.21037/atm.2018.12.14

Dairy:

https://www.mdpi.com/2072-6643/7/9/5339

https://www.tandfonline.com/doi/abs/10.1271/bbb.60267

https://www.ncbi.nlm.nih.gov/pmc/articles/PMC5041571/

https://www.ncbi.nlm.nih.gov/pmc/articles/PMC193670/

http://jjhres.com/en/articles/21863.html

220

Wheat and Gluten:

https://www.mdpi.com/2072-6643/5/3/771

https://www.ncbi.nlm.nih.gov/pubmed/23334113/

https://onlinelibrary.wiley.com/doi/full/10.1111/apt.12730

https://doi.org/10.1212/WNL.56.3.385

Alcohol:

https://www.ncbi.nlm.nih.gov/pmc/articles/PMC2828255/

https://www.ncbi.nlm.nih.gov/pmc/articles/PMC6339663/

https://www.karger.com/Article/Abstract/343908

High-AGE Foods:

See: Faloon, W. (2015). Live Longer by Changing How You Cook!. *Life Extension Magazine*, August 2015 issue.

Sugar:

https://www.lifeextension.com/magazine/2017/10/the-great-sugar-cover-up/page-01

https://academic.oup.com/ajcn/article/94/2/479/4597872

https://www.ncbi.nlm.nih.gov/pmc/articles/PMC6086430/

https://www.sciencedirect.com/science/article/abs/pii/S0165032718315040?via%3Dihub

What about Soy?

https://www.ncbi.nlm.nih.gov/pmc/articles/PMC5793271/

https://www.karger.com/Article/Fulltext/444735

http://www.bbc.com/future/story/20190816-is-soy-bad-for-womens-health

Infla-Menses

https://www.ncbi.nlm.nih.gov/pubmed/17474167

https://www.ncbi.nlm.nih.gov/pmc/articles/PMC5793271/

https://www.ncbi.nlm.nih.gov/pubmed/21745527/

https://www.ncbi.nlm.nih.gov/pmc/articles/PMC3982974/

https://www.ncbi.nlm.nih.gov/pmc/articles/PMC5188409/

https://www.honeycolony.com/article/lectin-levels-in-foods/

https://www.ecowatch.com/impossible-burger-gmo-soy-2637794276.html

Chronic Infections and Toxic Mould:

See: https://www.honeycolony.com/article/chronic-infections-busting-biofilms/

https://www.epa.gov/mold

http://www.mdpi.com/2072-6651/6/1/66/htm

https://www.9news.com.au/national/2018/04/30/11/59/mould-in-your-home-mp-calls-for-national-inquiry

https://www.survivingmold.com/mold-symptoms/understanding-the-illness

Dysbiosis and Leaky Gut:

Fredericks, G. (2019) The Longevity Microbiome: How Our Gut Ecosystem Affects Lifespan. *Nexus Magazine*, 26(4), 40-45.

https://doi.org/10.1093/humrep/17.7.1704

https://doi.org/10.1210/jc.2017-02153

EMF Exposure:

https://doi.org/10.3109/15368378.2015.1043357

https://link.springer.com/article/10.1007%2Fs10072-017-2850-8

Obesity:

http://doi.org/10.1093/ajcn/83.2.461S

http://diabetes.diabetesjournals.org/content/52/8/2097

https://journals.plos.org/plosone/article?id=10.1371/journal.pone.0134187

https://www.honeycolony.com/article/epigenetics/

https://medicalxpress.com/news/2019-08-ward-weight-gain-obesity-genes.html

https://www.ncbi.nlm.nih.gov/pmc/articles/PMC3279464/

Smoking:

https://doi.org/10.1289/ehp.001081019

https://www.ncbi.nlm.nih.gov/pubmed/25403655/

https://doi.org/10.1093/aje/kwn194

https://journals.plos.org/plosbiology/article?id=10.1371/journal.pbio.2003904

Toxins:

https://www.ncbi.nlm.nih.gov/pmc/articles/PMC3270432/

https://www.ncbi.nlm.nih.gov/pubmed/15703533

https://www.ncbi.nlm.nih.gov/pmc/articles/PMC4143889/

https://www.spandidos-publications.com/10.3892/ijmm.2016.2728

https://jneuroinflammation.biomedcentral.com/articles/10.1186/1742-2094-7-20

https://www.ncbi.nlm.nih.gov/pmc/articles/PMC3279464/

Seneff, S. (2019). *Glyphosate and Non-Hodgkin's Lymphoma*. Weston Price Foundation.

https://www.acnem.org/members/journals/ACNEM_Journal_June_2015.pdf

Alexandra Preston

Infla-Menses

https://doi.org/10.3390/e15041416

https://pdfs.semanticscholar.org/026b/28e31780f61aa36529e240672367291ad74
c.pdf

https://articles.mercola.com/sites/articles/archive/2019/02/13/absorbent-
hygiene-products-health-risks.aspx

https://www.sciencedirect.com/science/article/pii/S0890623818302259

Negative Emotions:

https://www.ncbi.nlm.nih.gov/pmc/articles/PMC2868080/

https://www.schoolofmagnificence.com.au/

https://www.ncbi.nlm.nih.gov/pubmed/14747646

https://www.researchgate.net/publication/297363623_From_menstrual_shame_t
o_bleeding_as_a_spiritual_practice_The_antecedents_of_menstruation_spiritualit
y_and_Australian_women's_experiences_of_transformation

What Can We Do About It?: Dietary Interventions

https://www.liebertpub.com/doi/10.1089/acm.2018.0340

A Plant-Based Diet:

http://doi.org/10.1002/clc.23027

https://www.foodnavigator.com/Article/2013/06/04/Vegetarians-have-
significantly-lower-mortality-rates-reveals-study

https://doi.org/10.3389/fimmu.2018.00908

https://www.ncbi.nlm.nih.gov/pmc/articles/PMC4245565/

https://medicalxpress.com/news/2017-06-vegetarian-diets-effective-body-
weight.html

http://doi.org/10.1093/humrep/deq044

https://www.sciencedirect.com/science/article/pii/S0029784499005256

https://www.sciencedirect.com/science/article/pii/S0009898112000423

https://academic.oup.com/aje/article/152/5/446/149515/

Preventing Deficiencies in a Plant-Based Diet:

https://www.ncbi.nlm.nih.gov/pmc/articles/PMC5622783/

https://www.ncbi.nlm.nih.gov/pmc/articles/PMC3999603/

https://www.dietitians.ca/Downloads/Factsheets/Food-Sources-of-Iron.aspx

https://vegetariannutrition.net/docs/Zinc-Vegetarian-Nutrition.pdf

https://www.ncbi.nlm.nih.gov/pmc/articles/PMC4571201/

https://doi.org/10.1371/journal.pone.0191887

https://www.ncbi.nlm.nih.gov/pubmed/12350079

https://www.researchgate.net/publication/11310851_Menaquinone-4_in_breast_milk_is_derived_from_dietary_phylloquinone

https://www.ncbi.nlm.nih.gov/pmc/articles/PMC4042564/

https://www.ncbi.nlm.nih.gov/pubmed/18992136

The Low-FODMAP Diet:

https://doi.org/10.1111/ajo.12594

The Ketogenic Diet:

https://charliefoundation.org/

https://www.ncbi.nlm.nih.gov/pmc/articles/PMC4124736/

https://www.ncbi.nlm.nih.gov/pmc/articles/PMC2716748/

https://www.ncbi.nlm.nih.gov/pmc/articles/PMC1334192/

Infla-Menses

The Paleo Diet:

https://doi.org/10.1002/oby.21815

https://www.medicaljournals.se/acta/content/html/10.2340/00015555-1358

https://drjockers.com/keto-carb-cycling-women/

Intermittent Fasting:

https://www.ncbi.nlm.nih.gov/pmc/articles/PMC6460288/

https://www.ncbi.nlm.nih.gov/pmc/articles/PMC5411330/

https://www.ncbi.nlm.nih.gov/pmc/articles/PMC6016225/

https://www.sciencedirect.com/science/article/pii/S0303720716304695

Going Organic:

http://altmedrev.com/archive/publications/15/1/4.pdf

https://blog.ecosia.org/ecosia-trees-senegal-agroforestry-agriculture/

Eat Your Fruit and Vegetables:

https://www.ncbi.nlm.nih.gov/pmc/articles/PMC6018917/

https://www.ncbi.nlm.nih.gov/pmc/articles/PMC6723319/

https://www.ncbi.nlm.nih.gov/pubmed/30538082/

https://www.leafscience.org/positive-results-from-urolithin-a-human-trial/

https://www.ncbi.nlm.nih.gov/pubmed/26458740

https://www.ncbi.nlm.nih.gov/pubmed/28619389

http://pages.jh.edu/jhumag/0408web/talalay.html

https://www.hindawi.com/journals/omcl/2016/5276130/

http://www.phcog.com/article.asp?issn=0973-1296;year=2015;volume=11;issue=44;spage=556;epage=563;aulast=Fard

https://www.hindawi.com/journals/mi/2015/720171/

https://link.springer.com/article/10.1007%2Fs13197-012-0859-9

https://www.sciencedirect.com/science/article/pii/S2213453016300362?via%3Dihub

https://www.hindawi.com/journals/ecam/2018/4128984/

https://www.ncbi.nlm.nih.gov/pubmed/21363935

https://www.ncbi.nlm.nih.gov/pmc/articles/PMC3012565/

https://www.ncbi.nlm.nih.gov/pubmed/31327131

Drink Your Tea:

https://www.hindawi.com/journals/ecam/2018/4128984/

https://journals.sagepub.com/doi/10.1177/1933719113488455

https://www.ncbi.nlm.nih.gov/pmc/articles/PMC4152895/

https://www.ncbi.nlm.nih.gov/pmc/articles/PMC6500245/

Chocolate Can Be Healthy:

https://www.greenmedinfo.health/blog/not-just-kids-adding-chocolate-milk-makes-it-healthier

https://www.ncbi.nlm.nih.gov/pmc/articles/PMC4696435/

https://blog.paleohacks.com/cacao-vs-cocoa/

Anti-Inflammatory Fatty Acids:

https://www.ncbi.nlm.nih.gov/pmc/articles/PMC3033240/

Infla-Menses

Braun, L., & Cohen, M. (2010). *Herbs and Natural Supplements: An Evidence-Based Guide* (3rd ed.). Churchill Livingstone Australia.

https://www.ncbi.nlm.nih.gov/pmc/articles/PMC3770499/

https://www.ncbi.nlm.nih.gov/pmc/articles/PMC2868080/

https://lpi.oregonstate.edu/mic/other-nutrients/essential-fatty-acids

http://doi.org/10.1016/j.ctim.2013.06.006

Probiotics and Fermented Foods:

https://link.springer.com/article/10.1007%2Fs10616-010-9326-5

https://www.lifeextension.com/magazine/2009/1/optimize-digestive-health/page-01

https://www.ncbi.nlm.nih.gov/pubmed/30662004

https://www.jstage.jst.go.jp/article/tjem/230/1/230_17/_html

https://www.ncbi.nlm.nih.gov/pmc/articles/PMC5859128/

Antioxidants:

https://www.hindawi.com/journals/omcl/2016/5276130/

http://doi.org/10.1186/1477-7827-7-54

https://www.ncbi.nlm.nih.gov/pmc/articles/PMC4359851/

https://www.ncbi.nlm.nih.gov/pmc/articles/PMC2077876/

Preston, A. (2014). *Nutritional Biochemistry Explained.* Lulu Press.

https://www.ncbi.nlm.nih.gov/pubmed/23737821

https://www.greenmedinfo.com/article/nac-can-be-used-substitute-insulin-sensitizing-agent-treatment-polycystic-ovar

B Vitamins:

228

https://www.ncbi.nlm.nih.gov/pmc/articles/PMC4869157/

https://www.ncbi.nlm.nih.gov/pmc/articles/PMC4359851

https://www.ncbi.nlm.nih.gov/pmc/articles/PMC2978275/

Vitamin D:

https://doi.org/10.1111/joim.12496

https://ncbi.nlm.nih.gov/pubmed/27147120

https://www.ncbi.nlm.nih.gov/pubmed/29447494

https://www.ncbi.nlm.nih.gov/pmc/articles/PMC6422848/

https://www.ncbi.nlm.nih.gov/pmc/articles/PMC6390422/

https://www.ncbi.nlm.nih.gov/pmc/articles/PMC3626048/

https://www.ncbi.nlm.nih.gov/pmc/articles/PMC5751189/

Minerals:

https://www.ncbi.nlm.nih.gov/pmc/articles/PMC4841933/

https://www.greenmedinfo.com/blog/magnesium-safe-first-line-defense-clinical-depression

https://www.ncbi.nlm.nih.gov/pmc/articles/PMC3626048/

https://www.ncbi.nlm.nih.gov/pubmed/17289285

https://www.ncbi.nlm.nih.gov/pubmed/25864256

https://www.ncbi.nlm.nih.gov/pubmed/26267328

What Can We Do About It?: Herbal Medicine

Trickey, R. (2011). *Women, hormones and the menstrual cycle.* Third edition. Trickey Enterprises.

Infla-Menses

http://europepmc.org/abstract/med/17879831

https://www.hindawi.com/journals/omcl/2016/5276130/

https://www.ncbi.nlm.nih.gov/pubmed/24439651

http://ircmj.com/en/articles/59647.html

https://www.ncbi.nlm.nih.gov/pmc/articles/PMC3964428/

https://www.ncbi.nlm.nih.gov/pmc/articles/PMC3611645/

https://www.ncbi.nlm.nih.gov/pmc/articles/PMC3877456/

https://www.ncbi.nlm.nih.gov/pubmed/16117603

https://academic.oup.com/painmedicine/article/16/12/2243/2460294

https://onlinelibrary.wiley.com/doi/abs/10.1002/ptr.5235

https://www.ncbi.nlm.nih.gov/pmc/articles/PMC4040198/

https://www.ncbi.nlm.nih.gov/pubmed/20834180

https://www.ncbi.nlm.nih.gov/pubmed/23735479

https://www.ncbi.nlm.nih.gov/pubmed/16029938

https://www.ncbi.nlm.nih.gov/pubmed/25866155

https://www.ncbi.nlm.nih.gov/pmc/articles/PMC3110835/

https://www.liebertpub.com/doi/10.1089/107555303321223035

https://www.ncbi.nlm.nih.gov/pmc/articles/PMC4775794/

https://www.sciencedirect.com/science/article/pii/S0378874113008246?via%3Dihub

https://www.ncbi.nlm.nih.gov/pubmed/26051565

https://www.hindawi.com/journals/ecam/2018/4128984/

https://www.ncbi.nlm.nih.gov/pmc/articles/PMC4152895/

https://doi.org/10.1016/j.bcp.2011.12.030

http://nopr.niscair.res.in/bitstream/123456789/3329/1/IJBB%2046%281%29%2059-65.pdf

https://www.ncbi.nlm.nih.gov/pmc/articles/PMC3941414/

https://www.ncbi.nlm.nih.gov/pubmed/26610378

https://www.hindawi.com/journals/omcl/2016/5276130/

https://www.ncbi.nlm.nih.gov/pubmed/30989923

https://florajournal.com/archives/2015/vol3issue3/PartA/3-1-9.1.pdf/

https://www.jaims.in/index.php/jaims/article/view/262/232

https://pdfs.semanticscholar.org/de54/db9710881015ce6a5006997ca07aadab8fc6.pdf

https://doi.org/10.4103/2225-4110.119723

https://www.ncbi.nlm.nih.gov/pmc/articles/PMC4649577/

https://doi.org/10.1371/journal.pone.0089566

https://www.ncbi.nlm.nih.gov/pmc/articles/PMC4624216/

https://www.ncbi.nlm.nih.gov/pmc/articles/PMC2972363/

See references at: Fallis, J. (2017). 25 Powerful Ways to Boost Your Endocannabinoid System, viewed 29 June 2019, https://www.optimallivingdynamics.com/blog/how-to-stimulate-and-support-your-endocannabinoid-system

https://www.ncbi.nlm.nih.gov/pmc/articles/PMC3165946/

https://bjsm.bmj.com/content/38/5/536

Infla-Menses
What Can We Do About It?: Lifestyle, Energy and Mindset

Stapleton, P., Porter, B., & Sheldon, T. (2013). *Quitting Smoking: How to Use Emotional Freedom Techniques.* International Journal of Healing and Caring.

Stapleton, P., Sheldon, T., & Porter, B. (2012). *Practical Application of Emotional Freedom Techniques for Food Cravings.* International Journal of Healing and Caring, 12(3).

https://journals.sagepub.com/doi/10.1177/0890117116661154

https://search.proquest.com/openview/9beab788618acb85a60c987badf33914/1?pq-origsite=gscholar&cbl=2034852

https://www.ncbi.nlm.nih.gov/pubmed/10794112

https://www.ncbi.nlm.nih.gov/pmc/articles/PMC5871310/

Noontil, A. (1994). *The Body is the Barometer of the Soul.* Acacia Ridge, QLD: Brumby Sunstate.

https://www.ncbi.nlm.nih.gov/pmc/articles/PMC5628565/

https://www.sbs.com.au/nitv/article/2019/10/02/traditional-aboriginal-healers-push-be-part-mainstream-healthcare

Elisabeth, R. (2018). *Diamond Matrix Masters Self-Mastery Level 1.* Balboa Press.

https://www.ncbi.nlm.nih.gov/pubmed/30901775

https://www.ncbi.nlm.nih.gov/pubmed/28187404

https://www.ncbi.nlm.nih.gov/pubmed/31434111

https://doi.org/10.4103/bfpt.bfpt_69_16

Doidge, N. (2017). *The Brain's Way of Healing.* Scribe Publications.

https://www.ncbi.nlm.nih.gov/pubmed/7531030

https://www.ncbi.nlm.nih.gov/pmc/articles/PMC4707291/

https://www.ncbi.nlm.nih.gov/pmc/articles/PMC2140080/

https://www.ncbi.nlm.nih.gov/pmc/articles/PMC2793346/

http://www.mdpi.com/1660-4601/14/4/368/htm

https://www.webmd.com/balance/features/negative-ions-create-positive-vibes#1

https://nutritionreview.org/2013/04/positive-health-benefits-negative-ions/

https://academic.oup.com/qjmed/article/92/4/193/1586500

http://siberiantimes.com/healthandlifestyle/others/news/like-ducks-to-water-in-the-snow-keeping-kids-healthy-siberian-style/

https://theconversation.com/health-check-why-swimming-in-the-sea-is-good-for-you-68583

https://www.scientificamerican.com/article/q-a-why-is-blue-light-before-bedtime-bad-for-sleep/

http://www.pnas.org/content/112/4/1232

https://www.ncbi.nlm.nih.gov/pubmed/29512136

https://www.ncbi.nlm.nih.gov/pubmed/29493042

https://www.ncbi.nlm.nih.gov/pubmed/29897261/

https://www.greenmedinfo.health/blog/research-confirms-sweating-detoxifies-dangerous-metals-petrochemicals

https://www.hindawi.com/journals/bmri/2017/3676089/

https://positivepsychologyprogram.com/self-determination-theory/

https://onlinelibrary.wiley.com/doi/full/10.1002/acr.21677